Handbook of
Home Hemodialysis

a LANGE medical book

Handbook of Home Hemodialysis

Editors

Daphne H. Knicely, MD, MEHP, FASN
Assistant Professor of Medicine
Department of Medicine/Division of Nephrology
Johns Hopkins University School of Medicine
Baltimore, Maryland

Emaad M. Abdel-Rahman, MD, PhD
Professor, Division of Nephrology, Department of Internal Medicine
Vice Chief, Division of Nephrology UVA
Division of Nephrology
University of Virginia Health System
Charlottesville, Virginia

Keiko I. Greenberg, MD, MHS
Assistant Professor of Medicine
Division of Nephrology and Hypertension
Medstar Georgetown University Hospital
Washington, DC

New York   Chicago   San Francisco   Athens   London   Madrid
Mexico City   New Delhi   Milan   Singapore   Sydney   Toronto

Handbook of Home Hemodialysis

1 2 3 4 5 6 7 8 9   LCR   25 24 23 22 21

ISBN 978-1-260-45863-3
MHID 1-260-45863-6

This book was set in TimesNRMT by MPS Limited.
The editors were Jason Malley and Kim J. Davis.
The production supervisor was Richard Ruzycka.
Project management was provided by Jyoti Shaw of MPS Limited.
The cover designer was W2 Design.

Library of Congress Cataloging-in-Publication Data

Names: Knicely, Daphne H., editor. | Abdel-Rahman, E. M., editor. | Greenberg, Keiko I., editor.
Title: Handbook of home hemodialysis / editors, Daphne H. Knicely, Emaad M. Abdel-Rahman, Keiko I. Greenberg.
Description: New York : McGraw Hill, [2021] | A LANGE medical book. | Includes bibliographical references and index. | Summary: "The *Handbook of Home Hemodialysis* was developed to serve as a resource that educates healthcare providers about home hemodialysis, provides in-depth instructions for implementing a home hemodialysis program, and ultimately gives more patients with end-stage kidney disease the opportunity to select home hemodialysis"-- Provided by publisher.
Identifiers: LCCN 2020038046 (print) | LCCN 2020038047 (ebook) | ISBN 9781260458633 (paperback) | ISBN 9781260458640 (ebook)
Subjects: MESH: Hemodialysis, Home
Classification: LCC RC901.7.H45 (print) | LCC RC901.7.H45 (ebook) | NLM WJ 378 | DDC 617.4/61059--dc23
LC record available at https://lccn.loc.gov/2020038046
LC ebook record available at https://lccn.loc.gov/2020038047

Contents

Chapter 1
Brief History of Home Hemodialysis 1
Sadichhya Lohani, MD and Daphne H. Knicely, MD, MEHP, FASN

Chapter 2
Patient Recruitment and Training
for Home Hemodialysis 13
Joel D. Glickman, MD and Rebecca Kurnik Seshasai, MD, MSHP

Chapter 3
Vascular Access for Home Hemodialysis 28
Anil K. Agarwal, MD, FACP, FASN, FNKF, FASDIN, Khaled Y. Boubes, MD, FASN, FASDIN, and Nabil F. Haddad, MD, FASDIN

Chapter 4
Prescribing Home Hemodialysis 44
Michael A. Kraus, MD, FACP and Michelle Carver, BSN, RN, CNN

Chapter 5
Water Handling in Home Hemodialysis 58
Keiko I. Greenberg, MD, MHS

Chapter 6
Laboratory Parameters and Monitoring
for Home Hemodialysis 69
Cynthia Christiano, MD and J. Clint Parker, MD, PhD

Contributors

Emaad M. Abdel-Rahman, MD, PhD
Professor, Division of Nephrology, Department of Internal Medicine
Vice Chief, Division of Nephrology UVA
Division of Nephrology
University of Virginia Health System
Charlottesville, Virginia
Chapter 8. Complications of Home Hemodialysis
Chapter 11. Quality of Life and Home Hemodialysis
Chapter 16. Remote Monitoring and Home Hemodialysis

Anil K. Agarwal, MD, FACP, FASN, FNKF, FASDIN
Professor of Medicine
Director of Interventional Nephrology
Section Chief of Nephrology at University Hospital East
The Ohio State University
Columbus, Ohio
Chapter 3. Vascular Access for Home Hemodialysis

Khaled Y. Boubes, MD, FASN, FASDIN
Assistant Professor of Medicine
The Ohio State University
Columbus, Ohio
Chapter 3. Vascular Access for Home Hemodialysis

Michelle Carver, BSN, RN, CNN
Vice President Clinical Service Home Therapy Initiatives
Fresenius Kidney Care
Waltham, Massachusetts
Chapter 4. Prescribing Home Hemodialysis

Christopher T. Chan, MD
Professor of Medicine
Division of Nephrology
University Health Network
Toronto, Ontario, Canada
Chapter 13. Special Populations and Home Hemodialysis

Alice Chedid, MD
Assistant Professor of Medicine
Department of Medicine/Division of Nephrology

University of Tennessee Health Science Center
Memphis, Tennessee
Chapter 7. Overview of Benefits and Limitations of Home Hemodialysis

Tushar Chopra, MD
Assistant Professor of Medicine/Nephrology
Department of Medicine/Division of Nephrology
University of Virginia
Charlottesville, Virginia
Chapter 8. Complications of Home Hemodialysis

Cynthia Christiano, MD
Associate Professor of Medicine
Division of Nephrology and HTN
Brody School of Medicine at East Carolina University
Greenville, North Carolina
Chapter 6. Laboratory Parameters and Monitoring for Home Hemodialysis

Michael Girsberger, MD
Division of Nephrology
University Health Network
Toronto, Ontario, Canada
Chapter 13. Special Populations and Home Hemodialysis

Joel D. Glickman, MD
Director, Home Dialysis Program
Professor of Clinical Medicine
Philadelphia, Pennsylvania
Chapter 2. Patient Recruitment and Training for Home Hemodialysis

Keiko I. Greenberg, MD, MHS
Assistant Professor of Medicine
Division of Nephrology and Hypertension
MedStar Georgetown University Hospital
Washington, DC
Chapter 5. Water Handling in Home Hemodialysis

Nupur Gupta, MD
Assistant Professor of Medicine
Indiana University Health
Indianapolis, Indiana
Chapter 15. Setting Up, Building, and Sustaining a Home Dialysis Program

Nabil F. Haddad, MD, FASDIN
Associate Professor of Medicine
The Ohio State University

Columbus, Ohio
Chapter 3. Vascular Access for Home Hemodialysis

Lakshmi Kannan, MBBS
Department of Medicine/Division of Nephrology
University of Virginia
Charlottesville, Virginia
Chapter 8. Complications of Home Hemodialysis

Daphne H. Knicely, MD, MEHP, FASN
Assistant Professor of Medicine
Department of Medicine/Division of Nephrology
Johns Hopkins University School of Medicine
Baltimore, Maryland
Chapter 1. Brief History of Home Hemodialysis
Chapter 7. Overview of Benefits and Limitations of Home Hemodialysis

Michael A. Kraus, MD, FACP
Associate Chief Medical Officer
Fresenius Kidney Care
Emeritus Professor of Clinical Medicine
Indiana University Medical Center
Fishers, Indiana
Chapter 4. Prescribing Home Hemodialysis
Chapter 14. Policy and Costs of Home Hemodialysis

Sadichhya Lohani, MD
Assistant Professor of Medicine
Renal Electrolyte and Hypertension
Penn Presbyterian Medical Center
Philadelphia, Pennsylvania
Chapter 1. Brief History of Home Hemodialysis

Brent W. Miller, MD
Professor of Medicine
Clinical Chief of Nephrology
Indiana University School of Medicine
Indianapolis, Indiana
Chapter 15. Setting Up, Building, and Sustaining a Home Dialysis Program

José A. Morfín, MD
Health Sciences Clinical Professor
Department of Internal Medicine, Nephrology Division
UC Davis School of Medicine
Sacramento, California
Chapter 9. Cardiovascular Outcomes and Home Hemodialysis

J. Clint Parker, MD, PhD
Assistant Professor of Medicine
Division of Nephrology and HTN
Brody School of Medicine at East Carolina University
Greenville, North Carolina
Chapter 6. Laboratory Parameters and Monitoring for Home Hemodialysis

Page V. Salenger, MD
Home Therapies Medical Director
Dialysis Clinic Inc.
Nashville, Tennessee
Chapter 10. Mineral Bone Disease in Home Hemodialysis

Rebecca Kurnik Seshasai, MD, MSHP
Assistant Professor of Clinical Medicine
University of Pennsylvania Perelman School of Medicine
Philadelphia, Pennsylvania
Chapter 2. Patient Recruitment and Training for Home Hemodialysis

Eric Weinhandl, PhD, MS
Senior Epidemiologist
Chronic Disease Research Group
Hennepin Healthcare Research Institute
Minneapolis, Minnesota
Chapter 12. Hospitalization and Home Hemodialysis
Chapter 14. Policy and Costs of Home Hemodialysis

Danielle Wentworth, MSN, FNP-BC
Division of Nephrology
University of Virginia
Charlottesville, Virginia
Chapter 16. Remote Monitoring and Home Hemodialysis

Nasim Wiegley, MD
Assistant Professor of Clinical Medicine
Department of Internal Medicine, Nephrology Division
UC Davis School of Medicine
Sacramento, California
Chapter 9. Cardiovascular Outcomes and Home Hemodialysis

Preface

Chronic kidney disease (CKD) is a prevalent condition associated with significant morbidity and mortality as well as considerable economic burden. A percentage of patients with CKD will eventually progress to end-stage kidney disease (ESKD) and require some form of dialysis. There are three dialysis options available; the large majority of patients opt for in-center hemodialysis (HD), with only a small proportion of patients performing peritoneal dialysis at home, and even fewer doing home hemodialysis (HHD). The predominance of in-center HD and underutilization of home dialysis modalities is likely related to what is offered to the patient, that is, healthcare providers have much more experience with in-center HD than with home modalities, and are much more comfortable referring patients for in-center HD.

When dialysis first became available, HHD was actually more prevalent than it is now. The proliferation of in-center HD units, which began in the 1970s, led to the decline in HHD. Due to the small size of the HHD population, nephrologists have limited exposure to HHD during training. Once they enter practice, nephrologists may not discuss HHD with patients due to a lack of knowledge about the modality. These days, healthcare providers frequently turn to online material or pocket guides to help them manage these gaps in knowledge. Through our research, we felt that there was a lack of texts about HHD. When it was discussed within a much larger context, the few pages devoted to HHD lacked the in-depth discussion necessary to truly manage a patient on HHD. We recognized this paucity of information as an opportunity to educate healthcare providers on this modality and to help build the HHD population.

The use of HHD in the United States has increased over the past 10 years. With new legislation, the Advancing American Kidney Health Initiative, introduced in the United States by the Department of Health and Human Services in July 2019, the number of HHD patients is expected to increase further. Home dialysis modalities provide more flexibility for patients. HHD is associated with benefits such as improved cardiovascular parameters and better quality of life. We need to provide patients with the chance to pursue these benefits if HHD fits with their lifestyle.

Our vision for the *Handbook of Home Hemodialysis* was to develop a resource that educates healthcare providers about HHD, provides in-depth instructions for implementing an HHD program, and ultimately gives more patients with ESKD the opportunity to select HHD. This book is not intended to be an all-encompassing text about HHD, but should provide healthcare providers a stepping off point to pursue further education through seminars, journals, and other resources. We hope that both nephrology trainees and established nephrologists can benefit from the *Handbook of Home Hemodialysis*.

Daphne H. Knicely, MD, MEHP, FASN
Emaad M. Abdel-Rahman, MD, PhD
Keiko I. Greenberg, MD, MHS

Dedication

To my husband, Kevin, thank you for all your support, encouragement, advice, and love. I am a better person because of you. To my girls, Ava and Mila, thank you for understanding that Mommy has to work sometimes. I do all of this for you. To my mother, Angela Harrington, who died of complications from end-stage kidney disease, you are the reason I am a nephrologist. I try to treat every patient as if he/she is family. Finally, to all my patients, you are the reason for this book. We wrote this book to help educate others, so they have more options to get you home.
—DHK

I would like to first dedicate this book to my Creator who gave me everything I have and to my parents, bless their souls. Would also like to dedicate it to my wife, my daughter, and my son who besides all their support helped me during the time I was dialyzing at home five times a week. The time I spent doing home hemodialysis taught me about end-stage kidney disease more than I learned being a nephrologist for more than 30 years. Not only did it allow me to identify with patients, but allowed me to understand more about care partners, my wife in my case who shouldered most of the burden. I hope this book will serve as a vehicle in teaching practicing nephrologist and trainees to better care of their patients and allowing patients to choose the best modality of care that matches their goals of life.
—EMAR

I dedicate this book to my family—my parents, sisters, husband, daughter, and extended family—for their constant support, encouragement, patience, and love. Thank you as well to my mentors, teachers, and colleagues, for shaping my medical education and making me the physician I am today. Most of all, I dedicate this book to the patients who have entrusted me with their care—helping you face the challenges of living with kidney disease is my honor and privilege.
—KIG

Abbreviations

AAMI	Association for the Advancement of Medical Instrumentation
ACE inhibitor	Angiotensin-converting enzyme inhibitor
Alk Phos	Alkaline phosphatase
ALT	Alanine aminotransferase
ANSI	American National Standards Institute
App	Application
ARB	Angiotensin-receptor blocker
ASN	American Society of Nephrology
AV	Arteriovenous
AVF	Arteriovenous fistula
AVG	Arteriovenous graft
BDI	Beck Depression Inventory
BUN	Blood urea nitrogen
BW	Body weight
CAD	Coronary artery disease
CaSRs	Calcium-sensing receptors
CfC	Conditions for Coverage
CFU	Colony-forming units
CHD	Conventional three times per week hemodialysis; thrice-weekly in-center hemodialysis; conventional hemodialysis
CKD	Chronic kidney disease
CLIMB study	Crit-Line Intradialytic Monitoring Benefit study

CMMI	Centers for Medicare and Medicaid Innovation
CMS	Centers for Medicare & Medicaid Services
CON	Certificate of Need
CPT	Current procedural terminology
CT	Computed tomography
CVC	Central venous catheter
CVD	Cardiovascular disease
DCC	Dialysate calcium concentration
DFC	Dialysis Facility Compare
DOPPS	Dialysis Outcomes and Practice Patterns Study
DRIP study	Dry Weight Reduction in Hypertensive Hemodialysis Patients study
EDW	Estimated dry weight
EEG	Electroencephalogram
EMS	Emergency medical services
EOD	Every other day
ESA	Erythropoietin-stimulating agent
ESKD	End-stage kidney disease
ESRD PPS	ESRD Prospective Payment System
ESRD QIP	ESRD Quality Incentive Program
EU	Endotoxin units
FDA	Food and Drug Administration
FGF-23	Fibroblast growth factor-23
FHN trial	Frequent Hemodialysis Network trial
FMLA	Family Medical Leave Act
FREEDOM	Following Rehabilitation, Economics, and Everyday-Dialysis Outcome Measurements
GFR	Glomerular filtration rate

HCV	Hepatitis C virus
HD	Hemodialysis
HF	Heart failure
HHD	Home hemodialysis
HHS	Health and Human Services
HIPAA	Health Insurance Portability and Accountability Act
HIV	Human immunodeficiency virus
HOMER-D	HOME Rehabilitation Treatment-Dialysis
HPT	Hyperparathyroidism
Hr-QOL	Health-related quality of life
HTN	Hypertension
ICD-10-CM	International Classification of Disease, 10th Edition, Clinical Modification
IDE	Investigational device exemption
IDH	Intradialytic hypotension
IDT	Interdisciplinary team
ISO	International Standards Organization
KDIGO	Kidney Disease: Improving Global Outcomes
KDOQI	Kidney Disease Outcomes Quality Initiative
KDQOL-36	Kidney disease quality of life 36-item short form survey
KEEP	Kidney Early Evaluation Program
LVEF	Left ventricular ejection fraction
LVH	Left ventricular hypertrophy
LVM	Left ventricular mass
MAC	Medicare Administrative Contractor
MAP	Mean arterial pressure
MBD	Mineral bone disorder/disease

MCP	Monthly capitated payment
MIPPA	Medicare Improvements for Patients and Providers Act
NHANES	National Health and Nutrition Examination Survey
NHD	Nocturnal hemodialysis
OSA	Obstructive sleep apnea
PAK	Purification pack
PCP	Primary care providers
PD	Peritoneal dialysis
PET	Positron emission tomography
PPPY	Per person per year
PTFE	Polytetrafluoroethylene
PTH	Parathyroid hormone
QA	Quality assurance
QAI	Quality assurance and improvement
QAPI	Quality assurance and process improvement
QOL	Quality of life
RO	Reverse osmosis
RPM	Remote patient monitoring
RRF	Residual renal function
RRT	Renal replacement therapy
RVUs	Relative value units
SCD	Sudden cardiac death
SDHD	Short daily hemodialysis
SF-36	Short form questionnaire-36 item
sp Kt/V	Single-pool Kt/V; non-equilibrated Kt/V
std Kt/V	Standard Kt/V; weekly standard Kt/V
TCU	Transitional care unit

TDC	Tunneled dialysis catheter
TVC	Total viable count
UF	Ultrafiltration
URR	Urea reduction ratio
USRDS	United States Renal Data System
VDRs	Vitamin D receptors

BRIEF HISTORY OF HOME HEMODIALYSIS 1

Sadichhya Lohani and Daphne H. Knicely

▌ BEGINNINGS OF HOME HEMODIALYSIS

The story of hemodialysis (HD) dates back to 1942 with the development of the first artificial kidney by Willem Kolff in Holland.[1,2] Italian Umberto Buoncristiani then built the first portable artificial kidney with recirculated dialysis fluid that enabled one of his patients to go on vacation with his children.[3] In Japan, HD was made available in 1954 by Kishuo Shibusawa who utilized the handmade, modified Skeggs hemodialyzer.[4] HD entered a new era when Belding Scribner and his colleagues from the University of Washington developed a Teflon arteriovenous shunt in 1960, making repeated blood access possible.[1,5] The first outpatient dialysis unit, the Seattle Artificial Kidney Center (now known as the Northwest Kidney Center), opened only 2 years later in 1962.[6] HD was only available for patients with acute kidney injury, who dialyzed 6 to 10 hours three times a week.[4] Home hemodialysis (HHD) was first established in the 1960s at the University of Washington in Seattle.[1]

In the early days of HD, given limited resources, there were ethical dilemmas regarding patient selection for HD. Later, in 1963, ethical concerns were raised surrounding the 15-year-old daughter of Albert Babb, who was a friend of Scribner. The young woman did not meet the criteria for in-center HD because of her age. At that time, Babb and Scribner were developing a proportioning HD unit used to make smaller single patient dialysis machines, which would be the precursor to modern-day HD machines.[1] In 1964, this HD equipment was used to perform the first HHD treatment—the patient was Albert Babb's daughter[1,7] (Figure 1-1).[4]

Even prior to 1964, there were independent efforts in various parts of the world to attempt HHD. In 1961, a Japanese patient was treated at home by using a coil dialyzer in an electric washing machine by Yukihiko Nose.[8] At that time, the electric washing machine was available in most homes in Japan. Thus, HD was mostly performed in patients' homes because the size of the machines made them difficult to transport.[4] With the help of a physician and an electric washing machine adapted for uremic blood, HD was done at home using the thoroughly cleaned electric washing machine (not sterilized) (Figure 1-2).[4] A disposable coil was suspended inside the washing machine by a strip of surgical bandage and, after establishing extracorporeal circulation, blood flows were monitored by a specially designed air bubble catcher. The standard dialysate powders, in batches, were packed separately as three components: electrolytes, bicarbonate, and glucose (Figure 1-3).[1] The powders were dissolved in 10 L of warm water and prepared inside the washing machine forming the resultant solution. If the patient's systolic blood pressure was more than 80 mm Hg, there

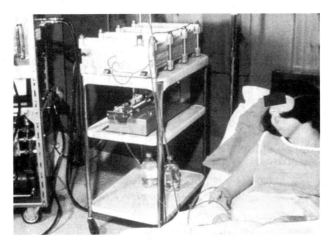

Figure 1-1 • The first home hemodialysis patient in Seattle, 1964. (*Reproduced with permission from Blagg CR. A brief history of home hemodialysis.* Adv Ren Replace Ther. *1996;3(2):99-105. Copyright © 1996 National Kidney Foundation. All rights reserved. Published by Elsevier Inc. All rights reserved. https://www.sciencedirect.com/journal/advances-in-renal-replacement-therapy.*)

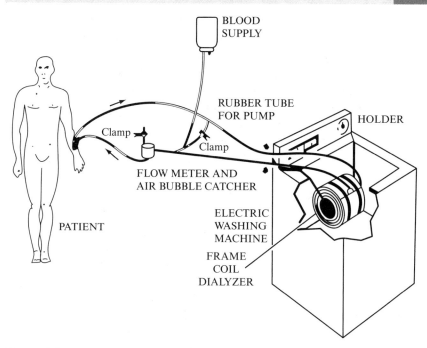

Figure 1-2 • Japanese home dialysis system with a frame coil dialyzer in an ordinary domestic washing machine. (*Reproduced with permission from Nosé Y. Home hemodialysis: A crazy idea in 1963: A memoir. ASAIO J. 2000;46(1):13-17. Copyright © by the American Society for Artificial Internal Organs. All rights reserved. https://journals.lww.com/asaiojournal/pages/default.aspx.*)

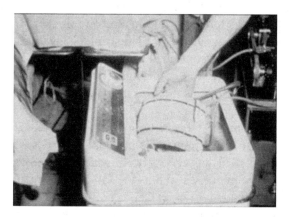

Figure 1-3 • The disposable coil dialyzer suspended inside a washing machine. (*Reproduced with permission from Nosé Y. Home hemodialysis: A crazy idea in 1963: A memoir. ASAIO J. 2000;46(1):13-17. Copyright © by the American Society for Artificial Internal Organs. All rights reserved. https://journals.lww.com/asaiojournal/pages/default.aspx.*)

was no need for a blood pump, but if necessary, a micrometer-driven roller pump was used. These pumps were run by eight standard 1.5-volt batteries for approximately 150 hours of use.[4] This HD technique was mainly used for patients with acute kidney injury and drug overdose.

When Yukihiko developed this technique of HHD, there was significant debate about the allocation of resources for HD in the United States. There were only a limited number of beds and dialyzers available for patients who needed HD. A committee at each HD unit determined which patients would receive chronic HD. Yukihiko came to the American Society for Artificial Internal Organs (ASAIO) Congress in Atlantic City in 1963 to present an abstract entitled "Hemodialysis at Home: Utilizing Domestic Electric Washing Machine." He proposed the use of the home washing machine for HHD with the thought that if patients were dialyzed at home, the need for such determinations of who could get HD would be avoided.[4]

In 1963, Scribner traveled to India to train a businessman on HHD.[1] During the same time, John Merrill used the twin-coil dialyzer to dialyze patients at home in Boston.[9] Also, Stanley Shaldon started an HHD program in London, and for the first time initiated nocturnal HHD with the availability of fail-safe monitoring for the HD machine.[1,10] These breakthroughs brought attention to HHD as an effective method of dialysis that was less expensive than conventional hemodialysis (CHD) as it did not require staff and could be done at home. The fail-safe monitoring system developed by Scribner and Shaldon became the foundation for all subsequent HHD machines.[1]

The development of HHD in the United Kingdom by Shaldon quickly triggered similar interest in France and Italy.[11] In 1965, both Scribner's group in Seattle and Merrill's group in Boston initiated HHD programs. Subsequently, HHD was offered at many centers, including Kolff's at the Cleveland Clinic.[4] Given continued limited availability of in-center HD, HD was done in patients' homes throughout the 1960s to 1970s, typically three times a week at night as this was more cost-effective than HD done at community units.[1,12,13]

Curtis et al. from the University of Washington reported their experience with the first HHD treatments in 1965. They described the use of the standard Seattle Kiil dialyzer, 3% acetic acid as the sterilizer, connecting tubes, sterilizing technique, as well as the fail-safe alarm system that was activated when the patient or caretaker were not awake. Patients and caretakers were trained for 2 months. The cost of the expendable material (dressings, heparin) was reported as $11 and monthly operating costs were $273.[7]

In 1967, the board of trustees of the Seattle Artificial Kidney Center Unit decided that all new patients started on HD must do HHD and that in-center HD patients should be encouraged to switch to HHD due to tremendous financial difficulties experienced by the unit. Scribner opened a training center for HHD at the University of Washington's Coach House dialysis facility in a local motel.[1] Patients from Seattle and from across the United States and abroad came to receive HHD training at this unit during the 1960s.[1,14] Because of the training provided at this center, more than 90% of dialysis patients in western Washington were on HHD by the 1970s.[1] They also developed video-based training to facilitate shortening of training time.[1,15]

HHD continued to be increasingly used in the early era of dialysis because of its multiple advantages over in-center HD, including cost-effectiveness, ability to avoid onerous travel to reach a dialysis unit, lower infection risk, and increased rehabilitation and independence. Hence by 1973, when the Medicare End-Stage Renal Disease (ESRD) program began, approximately 32.3% patients with end-stage kidney disease (ESKD) in the United States were on HHD.[1] In Australia and New Zealand also, more than half of the HD population was treated at home in the 1970s to 1980s.[16]

▍DECLINE OF HOME HEMODIALYSIS

The Medicare ESRD program established in 1972 provided nearly universal coverage for dialysis and transplantation.[1,17–19] In the same year, Australia introduced universal health coverage providing free care for all dialysis modalities and regimens both in-center and at home.[20] Improved funding for dialysis led to the development of more in-center HD units as well as the emergence of for-profit dialysis units. This coupled with decreased funding for HHD between 1973 and 1978, aging and increasing medical complexity of the ESKD population, and patient preference to dialyze at in-center units due to the convenience of having staff manage their dialysis treatments led to increasing popularity of in-center HD.[1,3,17,21]

The extensive training and complexity of HHD, need for an extensive support system, equipment maintenance, lack of adequate supplies, and lack of nephrologist experience in HHD all contributed to significant decline in HHD.[1] HHD training required dedication and time from the nursing staff, patient, and care partner; the lack of trained staff, caretakers, and support systems was a significant hindrance to HHD. Some facilities would not allow HHD without a partner or a care partner being available to assist the patient in the event of an emergency during treatments at home.[21] In addition, some countries raised concerns about the legal ramifications of HD complications occurring in the absence of direct physician supervision during treatment.[21] These factors played a role in the gradual loss of enthusiasm among providers and patients for HHD.[17]

Another factor that led to the decline in HHD was the growth of kidney transplant due to increased eligibility of non related donors and expanded inclusion criteria for cadaveric donors. As patients on HHD were highly motivated patients with lower disease burden compared to those on in-center HD, they were ideal candidates for transplantation. As more HHD patients received transplants, the proportion of ESKD patients on HHD further declined.[21] During the same period, peritoneal dialysis (PD) emerged as a modality with the development of the implantable Tenckhoff peritoneal catheter in 1968.[22] A safe and affordable discard system made PD more lucrative for physicians and attractive to patients interested in a home modality.[1,16]

With the decline in the proportion of patients on HHD during the 1970s, only 4.6% of patients on dialysis were on HHD by the 1980s.[1] In Washington, where 90% of patients had been on HHD in the 1960s, only 11.4% remained on HHD at the end of 1994. By December 2005, only 0.58% (2105 out of 341,319) of all ESKD patients on dialysis were on HHD in the United States.[17,23] In the early 2000s, only Australia, New Zealand, and Turkey reported significant use of HHD (about 11.1%, 13.7%, and 11.1%, respectively).[21,24] Most recently, only the United Kingdom, New Zealand, and Australia have been able to maintain significant numbers of patients on HHD. In Australia, the main driver for continued HHD use has been geography—some patients must travel hundreds of kilometers to reach the nearest dialysis unit.[21]

Despite decreasing use of HHD in the United States, efforts to maintain HHD continued in Seattle —this included the provision of paid aides to help patients with treatments, which was supported by Health Care Financing Administration funding. In 1983, Congress introduced composite rate reimbursement with equal payment for in-center and HHD and excluded payment for aides for HHD.[1]

▌RESURGENCE OF HOME HEMODIALYSIS

After decades of decline, HHD has seen a resurgence since 2000 due to improved outcomes related to frequent HD, cost-effectiveness of HHD, and availability of simpler, more portable, and safer HHD equipment.

Favorable Clinical Outcomes

In the 1960s, HD was done only on an as-needed basis for life-threatening indications or uremic symptoms. HD frequency was gradually increased from once or twice a week as it became evident that such regimens were inadequate. Eventually, the frequency became standardized at three times a week, although daily dialysis was being studied in California as early as 1967.[25] Consideration of more frequent HD was limited as the number of patients rose, and dialysis units filled.[26]

At the ASAIO annual meeting in 1995, there was discussion about building new HHD equipment that could be readily and safely used at home.[1] At the same conference, John Woods and his colleagues reported improved survival of ESKD patients on HHD compared to CHD.[27] In 1996, Robert Uldall first described slow nocturnal HHD in six patients in a Toronto hospital, dialyzing with a central venous catheter for 8 hours overnight up to six nights a week with blood flow rates of 300 mL/min and dialysate flow rates of 100 mL/min.[28] They reported significant improvement in patient outcomes, including improved Kt/V, improved blood pressure leading to discontinuation of anti hypertensive medications, better phosphorus control, better energy, improved sleep, and improved functional status.[28] Subsequently in 1998, another study by Pierratos et al. showed similar benefits in clinical outcomes, including improved blood pressure, phosphorus control, and functional status with nocturnal HHD with lower overall cost.[29]

The Frequent Hemodialysis Network (FHN) Trial, which compared patients randomized to six times per week (in-center short daily or nocturnal HHD) or three times per week HD, reported that the short daily group was found to have a lower risk of the composite outcome of death or increase in left ventricular (LV) mass.[30] Similar benefits were seen in studies out of Canada and Australia which favored frequent nocturnal hemodialysis (NHD).[31,32] Mortality benefit was seen in a retrospective multicenter study by Rivara et al. examining extended hours of HD.[33] Buchanan et al. also proposed that the major determinant of intradialytic cardiac stunning was volume removal and ultrafiltration (UF) rate.[34] Thus, the extended hours of HHD allowed for slower UF rates, minimizing cardiac stunning.[21,35] HHD also provided flexibility and independence for patients, and avoided the long weekend break from dialysis.[21,32,36]

These studies revived interest in HHD. As more patient-friendly systems for HD were developed, the proportion of HHD patients started to gradually increase.[17] The cost-effectiveness of HHD has also prompted increased use.[21]

[For more information, see Chapters 7, 9, 10, and 11.]

Cost-Effectiveness

The cost-effectiveness of HHD has been studied. Nocturnal and daily home therapy provided three times greater treatment time on HD at one-fifth lower cost in Canada, 11% cost savings in an Australian cohort, and financial advantages with daily HD in the United States. These cost advantages were due to decreased labor costs, lower hospital admissions, and decreased medication requirements.[12,37–39] The durable HHD equipment, which can last up to 10 years, has been noted to be less expensive overall compared to the overall cost for in-center HD.[21]

[For more information, see Chapters 12 and 14.]

Promising Technology

The Aksys Personal Hemodialysis System was the first patient-friendly HHD equipment (PHDTM; Lincolnshire, IL, USA). Developed in the early 1990s, it was designed for short daily HHD.[17,40] This machine was withdrawn in 2006 due to financial issues.[17] Then, in 2005, NxStage Medical, Inc. (Lawrence, MA, USA) launched a much smaller HHD device called the System One onto the market—this used 20 L or more of dialysate in 5 L premixed bags.[17,41] Subsequently, the PureFlow system was developed to be used with the NxStage System One. This device purifies water and produces up to 60 L of dialysate, enough for one to three dialysis sessions, at a time.[17] Another small company, Renal Solutions, Inc. (Warrendale, PA, USA) also developed a sorbent-based system, the Allient, for HHD. It uses a cartridge containing activated charcoal and zirconium resins to absorb toxins and requires only a few liters of water for dialysis.[17,42] NxStage and Renal Solutions were later acquired by Fresenius Medical Care.[17] Safety measures were also under development, including the use of pre-perforated dialysis catheter caps and moisture sensors to detect disconnections.[29]

HHD machines have become more streamlined over time, with more efficient and quiet water treatment systems, simpler control panels on machines, and simpler setup for the cartridge-based lines.[21] In the United States, the introduction of the portable NxStage machine with its simple on-off switch and quick operating procedure had a major impact on promoting and expanding HHD.[20,41] Several other home-friendly machines have been developed recently, including the Quanta, Physidia, and C-PAK machines. The availability of communication technologies has made it easier to monitor home treatments, recording and transmitting information including blood pressure, weight, treatment details, and alarms.[20] In the United States, Medicare will now pay for a monthly comprehensive televisit with the patient that originates from his/her home or a dialysis unit without geographic restrictions.[43] The availability of these technologies has made HHD more convenient for providers as well as patients. These technologies, however, should be used carefully to avoid excessive intrusiveness of healthcare providers into patients' lives.[44]

[For more information, see Chapter 16.]

▌RECENT TRENDS IN HOME HEMODIALYSIS

In the past decade, there have been some positive trends in HHD in the United States, resulting in an increased use of HHD. In this period, aided by the increasing popularity of the NxStage family of HD systems, the US HHD population has more than tripled from about 0.4% to about 1.5% of all patients on dialysis.[3] By 2015, there were more than 5000 HHD patients in the United States.[45] The trend is expected to continue as the number of dialysis patients increase out of proportion to the dialysis center capacity and staff.[21] The increasing number of studies and experiences have continued to show improved outcomes and subsequent cost reduction with HHD, creating enthusiasm and renewed interest among nephrologists. This promising trend has been seen worldwide, even in countries such as Australia and New Zealand where a significant proportion of patients were already on HHD.[21] At the end of 2017, about 18% of all dialysis patients in Australia and 47% in New Zealand were dialyzing at home.[46] Australia and New Zealand's HHD regimens favor long, slow, frequent, and NHD, while the short daily home regimens are favored in the United States.[3] Some countries such as Australia have even started to provide incentives to HHD programs and financial assistance to patients who choose HHD.[21,47] Despite the recent increase in the number of HHD patients in the United States, the overall utilization of HHD remains very low. At the end of 2017, 98% of HD patients were dialyzed at a center and only 2.0% dialyzed at home.[48] The trend of in-center HD and HHD is summarized in Figure 1-4.[49]

▌FUTURE OF HOME HEMODIALYSIS

Several newer systems are emerging that favor home and/or self-care, and aim to meet patient demand for more portable systems.[3] Smaller HHD systems are being developed, including the Home Hemodialysis Plus Vera (Home Hemodialysis Plus, Portland, OR, USA), which uses a new, very small dialyzer. Wearable artificial kidneys are also in development.[17,50] This soon will further change the landscape of HHD for the next generation.

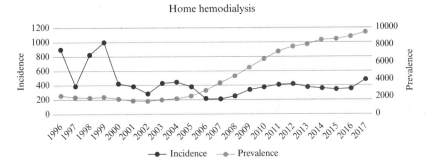

Figure 1-4 • Trend of incident counts and prevalent counts of ESKD on home hemodialysis 1996 to 2017 (USRDS 2019). The prevalence of home hemodialysis has increased over time. The number of new ESKD patients per year who opt for home hemodialysis has declined since the 1990s reflecting the shift toward in-center dialysis. The increased prevalence of home hemodialysis since 2005 reflects the launch of the NxStage home hemodialysis machines. (*The data reported here was supplied by the United States Renal Data System [USRDS]. The interpretation and reporting of this data is the responsibility of the authors and in no way should be seen as an official policy or interpretation of the US government.*)

▋REFERENCES

1. Blagg CR. A brief history of home hemodialysis. *Adv Ren Replace Ther.* 1996;3(2):99-105.
2. Kolff WJ. First clinical experience with the artificial kidney. *Ann Intern Med.* 1965;62:608-619.
3. Agar JWM, Barraclough KA, Piccoli GB. Home haemodialysis: how it began, where it went wrong, and what it may yet be. *J Nephrol.* 2019;32(3):331-333.
4. Nose Y. Home hemodialysis: a crazy idea in 1963: a memoir. *ASAIO J.* 2000;46(1):13-17.
5. Quinton W, Dillard D, Scribner BH. Cannulation of blood vessels for prolonged hemodialysis. *Trans Am Soc Artif Intern Organs.* 1960;6:104-113.
6. Haviland JW. Experiences in establishing a community artificial kidney center. *Trans Am Clin Climatol Assoc.* 1966;77:125-136.
7. Curtis FK, Cole JJ, Tyler LL, Scribner BH. Hemodialysis in the home. *Trans Am Soc Artif Intern Organs.* 1965;11:7-10.
8. Nose Y, Topaz S, Sengupta A, et al. Artificial hearts inside the pericardial sac in calves. *Trans Am Soc Artif Intern Organs.* 1965;11:255-262.
9. Merrill JP. Hemodialysis in the home. *JAMA.* 1968;206(1):124.
10. Baillod RA, Comty C, Ilahi M, et al. Overnight haemodialysis in the home. *Proc Eur Dial Transplant Assoc.* 1965;2:99-103.
11. Shaldon S. History of home hemodialysis. *J Nephrol.* 2004;17(2):316-317.
12. Trinh E, Chan CT. The rise, fall, and resurgence of home hemodialysis. *Semin Dial.* 2017;30(2):174-180.
13. Young BA, Chan C, Blagg C, et al. How to overcome barriers and establish a successful home HD program. *Clin J Am Soc Nephrol.* 2012;7(12):2023-2032.

14. Blagg CR, Hickman RO, Eschbach JW, et al. Home hemodialysis: six years' experience. *N Engl J Med*. 1970;283(21):1126-1131.
15. Stinson GW, Clark MF, Sawyer TK, et al. Home hemodialysis training in 3 weeks. *Trans Am Soc Artif Intern Organs*. 1972;18(0):66-69.
16. Agar JW. International variations and trends in home hemodialysis. *Adv Chronic Kidney Dis*. 2009;16(3):205-214.
17. Blagg CR. The renaissance of home hemodialysis: where we are, why we got here, what is happening in the United States and elsewhere. *Hemodial Int*. 2008;12(suppl 1):S2-S5.
18. Institute of Medicine (US) Committee to study decision making. In: Hanna KE, ed. *Biomedical Politics*. Washington, DC: National Academies Press; 1991. Origins of the Medicare Kidney Disease Entitlement: The Social Security Amendments of 1972.
19. Retting RA, Marks E. *Implementing the End-Stage Renal Disease Program of Medicare*. Publication R-2505-HCFA/HEW. Santa Monica, CA: The Rand Corporation; 1980:191-212.
20. Ing TS, Rahman MA, Kjellstrand CM. *Dialysis: History, Development and Promise*. Singapore: World Scientific; 2012.
21. Kerr PG, Jaw J. Home hemodialysis: what is old is new again. In: La Manna G, Ronco C, eds. *Contributions to Nephrology*. Vol 190. Basel: Karger AG; 2017:146-155.
22. Tenckhoff H, Schechter H. A bacteriologically safe peritoneal access device. *Trans Am Soc Artif Intern Organs*. 1968;14:181-187.
23. United States Renal Data System. USRDS 2007 annual data report: atlas of chronic kidney disease and end-stage renal disease in the United States. National Institutes of Health, National Institute of Diabetes and Digestive and Kidney Diseases, Bethesda, MD; 2007.
24. United States Renal Data System. USRDS 2003 annual data report: atlas of end-stage renal disease in the United States. National Institutes of Health, National Institute of Diabetes and Digestive and Kidney Diseases, Bethesda, MD; 2003.
25. DePalma JR, Pecker EA, Maxwell MH. A new automatic coil dialyzer system for "daily" dialysis. *Hemodial Int*. 2004;8(1):19-23.
26. Kjellstrand CM. A brief history of daily hemodialysis. *Home Hemodial Int*. 1998;2(1):8-11.
27. Woods JD, Port FK, Stannard D, et al. Comparison of mortality with home hemodialysis and center hemodialysis: a national study. *Kidney Int*. 1996;49(5):1464-1470.
28. Uldall R, Ouwendyk M, Francoeur R, et al. Slow nocturnal home hemodialysis at the Wellesley Hospital. *Adv Ren Replace Ther*. 1996;3(2):133-136.
29. Pierratos A, Ouwendyk M, Francoeur R, et al. Nocturnal hemodialysis: three-year experience. *J Am Soc Nephrol*. 1998;9(5):859-868.
30. Chertow GM, Levin NW, Beck GJ, et al. In-center hemodialysis six times per week versus three times per week. *N Engl J Med*. 2010;363(24):2287-2300.
31. Pauly RP, Maximova K, Coppens J, et al. Patient and technique survival among a Canadian multicenter nocturnal home hemodialysis cohort. *Clin J Am Soc Nephrol*. 2010;5(10):1815-1820.

32. Jun M, Jardine MJ, Gray N, et al. Outcomes of extended-hours hemodialysis performed predominantly at home. *Am J Kidney Dis.* 2013;61(2):247-253.

33. Rivara MB, Adams SV, Kuttykrishnan S, et al. Extended-hours hemodialysis is associated with lower mortality risk in patients with end-stage renal disease. *Kidney Int.* 2016;90(6):1312-1320.

34. Buchanan C, Mohammed A, Cox E, et al. Intradialytic cardiac magnetic resonance imaging to assess cardiovascular responses in a short-term trial of hemodiafiltration and hemodialysis. *J Am Soc Nephrol.* 2017;28(4):1269-1277.

35. Jefferies HJ, Virk B, Schiller B, et al. Frequent hemodialysis schedules are associated with reduced levels of dialysis-induced cardiac injury (myocardial stunning). *Clin J Am Soc Nephrol.* 2011;6(6):1326-1332.

36. Liu J, Foley RN. Alternate-day dialysis may be needed for hemodialysis patients. *Kidney Int.* 2012;81(11):1055-1057.

37. McFarlane PA, Pierratos A, Redelmeier DA. Cost savings of home nocturnal versus conventional in-center hemodialysis. *Kidney Int.* 2002;62(6):2216-2222.

38. Agar JW, Knight RJ, Simmonds RE, et al. Nocturnal haemodialysis: an Australian cost comparison with conventional satellite haemodialysis. *Nephrology.* 2005;10(6):557-570.

39. Mohr PE, Neumann PJ, Franco SJ, et al. The case for daily dialysis: its impact on costs and quality of life. *Am J Kidney Dis.* 2001;37(4):777-789.

40. Kjellstrand CM, Blagg CR, Bower J, et al. The Aksys personal hemodialysis system. *Semin Dial.* 2004;17(2):151-153.

41. Clark WR, Turk JE Jr. The NxStage System One. *Semin Dial.* 2004;17(2):167-170.

42. Ash SR. The Allient dialysis system. *Semin Dial.* 2004;17(2):164-166.

43. Lew SQ, Sikka N. Operationalizing Telehealth for home dialysis patients in the United States. *Am J Kidney Dis.* 2019;74(1):95-100.

44. Rajkomar A, Farrington K, Mayer A, et al. Patients' and carers' experiences of interacting with home haemodialysis technology: implications for quality and safety. *BMC Nephrol.* 2014;15:195.

45. United States Renal Data System. 2015 USRDS annual data report: epidemiology of kidney disease in the United States. National Institutes of Health, National Institute of Diabetes and Digestive and Kidney Diseases, Bethesda, MD; 2015.

46. ANZDATA: Annual Report 2018. 2019.

47. Klag MJ, Whelton PK, Randall BL, et al. Blood pressure and end-stage renal disease in men. *N Engl J Med.* 1996;334(1):13-18.

48. United States Renal Data System. 2018 USRDS annual data report: Chapter 1. Incidence, prevalence, patient characteristics, and treatment modalities. National Institutes of Health, National Institute of Diabetes and Digestive and Kidney Diseases, Bethesda, MD; 2018.

49. United States Renal Data System. 2019 USRDS annual data report: epidemiology of kidney disease in the United States. National Institutes of Health, National Institute of Diabetes and Digestive and Kidney Diseases, Bethesda, MD; 2019.

50. Davenport A, Gura V, Ronco C, et al. A wearable haemodialysis device for patients with end-stage renal failure: a pilot study. *Lancet.* 2007;370(9604):2005-2010.

PATIENT RECRUITMENT AND TRAINING FOR HOME HEMODIALYSIS

2

Joel D. Glickman and Rebecca Kurnik Seshasai

Although it has been said that patients choose home hemodialysis (HHD) because they feel better and achieve better outcomes, in reality they cannot appreciate those benefits before they start HHD. Therefore, it is more likely that most patients choose HHD because they aspire to enjoy a better quality of life (QOL). Patients continue on HHD therapy because their perceived benefit outweighs their obligate burden of performing HHD at home. The burden begins with making the difficult decision to take on the responsibility of performing HHD. The home dialysis staff needs to ensure that during the modality education period, patients receive sufficient time and support to mitigate the stress of choosing the best dialysis modality that will enable them to realize their life plans. The staff also needs to be certain that patients have appropriate skills, home environment, and support to succeed on HHD. Plans must be made to correct modifiable barriers for success. Unmodifiable barriers must be identified, recognized, and explained to the patient who is not suitable for HHD.

The burden of training for HHD should not be underestimated. It requires a significant time commitment on behalf of the patient and, if pertinent, the care partner. Learning new terminologies and procedures that in all likelihood are very foreign to the patient and partner is very stressful. However, the training period is also an opportunity to improve patient benefit and decrease the burden of therapy. The home dialysis team has the undivided attention of the patient and therefore can develop a personal and trusting relationship. The staff has the opportunity to learn more about the patient's home environment, daily schedule, and life plans that will help inform decisions regarding a preferred treatment duration and schedule. Learning more about the patient's personality, perceived strengths, and fears will help the staff understand how to relate better to patient needs.

Fundamental to successful relationships between staff and patients is communication. It is only effective if the participants agree to nonjudgmental, unconditional, and mutually respectful communication. That is to say, patients should feel comfortable enough to tell healthcare providers about any problems, errors, and concerns without fear of reprimand for not following instructions or plans, or fear that they will not be heard and problems will be dismissed. The staff must assure the patient that the focus of the program is the patient and that the staff is only concerned about their health, safety, and well-being. They also need to guarantee that patient complaints will be acknowledged and validated, and that if a solution cannot be provided, other healthcare providers will be consulted. However, the patient needs to understand that at times they may need to receive constructive feedback that is aimed to optimize their treatment and achieve the best outcomes possible.

▌THE "IDEAL PATIENT"

There are different ways to define the "ideal patient." It could be the patient who would most benefit from the medical advantages of HHD compared to in-center hemodialysis (HD). For a new HHD program about to train its first patient, it might be the patient who has significant partner support, is very knowledgeable about HD and their own treatment, and can self-cannulate already. From the patient perspective, those with a demanding and inflexible work schedule, a family member at home who needs daily attention, or a desire to travel might find HHD to be an ideal therapy. In general, the ideal patient is highly motivated and strongly desires to do dialysis at home.

Patients who would most benefit from more frequent HHD may have difficult-to-control hypertension, struggle with volume control, chronic hyperphosphatemia, left ventricular hypertrophy, decreased cardiac ejection fraction, or have contraindications to peritoneal dialysis (PD) but the desire to continue on a home therapy. Some younger patients may have contraindications for transplant because of non modifiable factors (e.g., recurrent renal disease after prior renal transplant, or anatomic abnormalities). We recommend more frequent HD, especially nocturnal hemodialysis (NHD), for these patients to hopefully improve long-term survival.

Patients with disabilities should also have the opportunity to benefit from HHD therapy. Caring for disabled patients may pose additional challenges, which will require innovative solutions by the home dialysis staff. As is true for all HHD patients, care needs to be individualized and based on the abilities and circumstances of the individual patient. Problem solving to accommodate patients with disability will take extra commitment and, at times, "out-of-the-box" thinking.

There are contraindications to HHD that include patients and/or partners who are unable to make appropriate decisions or follow instructions, have significant psychiatric or neurologic disease including dementia, chronically use sedating medications or illicit drugs, or have an access that is unsuitable for self-cannulation.

[For more information, see Chapters 7, 9, and 10.]

▌THE TRAINER

The trainer nurse must be an outstanding communicator and educator, and also a very proficient HD nurse. If the HHD program is not large enough to support more than one nurse, the trainer will also need to manage day-to-day issues and monthly clinic visits for the other HHD patients in the clinic. In larger programs with multiple nurses, it is ideal to have one expert trainer who has the most experience but all the nurses should be completely competent to train a patient. The trainer will need to be trained by the dialysis provider, but it will take support from other trained HHD nurses in order to become a skilled trainer who can manage patients with challenging circumstances. It is essential in any program to have all the trainers follow the exact same procedures and policies in order to prevent any inconsistencies that may lead to confusion on the part of the patient.

[For more information, see Chapter 15.]

▌PATIENT RECRUITMENT

Patients need education regarding dialysis modality options regardless of their position in the chronic kidney disease (CKD) continuum. HHD should be offered as an option to both incident and prevalent dialysis patients. Patients with CKD stage G4 and G5 should attend at least one, but preferably several, CKD education classes. When exposed to a good CKD education program, about 8% of patients will choose HHD.[1,2] Patients with failing kidney transplants as well as patients with CKD because of other solid organ transplants tend to be highly motivated patients and are excellent candidates for HHD. It is imperative to develop a relationship with transplant programs to make sure their patients receive adequate instruction regarding the benefits of HHD.

Similarly, PD patients who need to transfer to HD are often very interested in HHD. If the HHD program is located in the same space as a PD program the staff should work together to help patients continue home dialysis treatments if they so desire.

Even in acute start dialysis situations, modality education will be able to successfully recruit patients. In one study, approximately 10% of acute start dialysis patients eventually performed HHD after exposure to an in-hospital CKD education program.[3]

▌SCREENING EVALUATION

The training process is long and requires significant time, effort, and expense for the patient, HHD staff, and dialysis provider. Therefore, it is extremely important to ensure that the decision to start training is the appropriate decision. If the screening process is overly lax, then patients and staff may become disappointed and frustrated because training is not successful. On the other hand, excessively strict criteria may miss the "diamond in the rough" who would flourish on HHD. As a program becomes more experienced, the screening process can become more nuanced and productive.

It is essential to have a comprehensive and informative session with the patient prior to starting HHD. The staff should not hear from a patient during or nearing the end of training "you never told me I needed to do that; I don't think I can." The screening process should include an initial phone call, extended patient visit to the HHD clinic in order to meet with the multidisciplinary team, and finally an HHD staff visit to the patient's home. Hopefully, the patient has had adequate modality education prior to referral and has some knowledge about HHD. In cases where the patient has not been adequately informed, modality education must be provided before starting screening. In a one-to-one modality education session, sometimes basic screening can be done at the same time.

The first step in screening is a phone call meant to determine if basic program requirements are met. During a relatively brief but organized phone call, the staff can determine fairly accurately if patients will not succeed on HHD. The patient should have realistic reasons and goals for doing HHD and there should be no insurmountable obstacles. First and foremost, the potential HHD patient should be interested and motivated to perform HHD. If a patient's only reason for doing HHD is "my doctor thought it would be a good idea," then there is a very good chance the patient will not be suitably engaged to succeed on HHD. On the other hand, if the patient wants better outcomes, dialysis schedule flexibility, active involvement in their care, more free time for work or family, and the opportunity to travel, they are much more likely to thrive on HHD. The staff must explain in detail the extensive training schedule as well as the time commitment needed to correctly perform HHD. If the patient does not understand and cannot commit, then a follow-up phone call or meeting with the HHD team in the clinic facility should be scheduled to repeat the discussion. There may be factors that absolutely preclude HHD such as lack of a permanent or stable residence, significant physical ailments and limitations, and drug or alcohol addiction. If patients do not qualify after the initial screening, then they need to be told why. If there are factors that can be corrected, the staff should provide advice and counseling, and offer the patient a follow-up screening call or a face-to-face meeting. However, if there are factors that cannot be corrected, it should be clearly explained to the patient.

Interested patients should then have an in-person screening evaluation by the HHD care team, including the physician, nurse, dietitian, and social worker. The overarching goal is to determine whether the patient, and care partner if there is one, will be able to successfully provide dialysis therapy in the home setting while following all procedures to guarantee patient safety. Although discussed during the screening phone call, it is useful to once again ask patients why they are interested in HHD, what they already know about the training period and performing dialysis at home, and what their lifestyle is like (do they work, care for family members, travel, go to school, etc.).

The in-person meeting should include five broad subjects:

1. Home environment
2. Supplies and equipment
3. Patient cognitive and psychosocial status and physical skill set
4. Patient and care partner expectations
5. Detailed medical information

Given that the home will become a "medical facility," the home environment must be prepared to accommodate home dialysis treatments, but at the same time HHD should not overburden the home space and infrastructure. Setting up a dialysis facility in the home and managing supplies can be very obtrusive and the staff needs to ensure that the patient understands and agrees that all the requirements can be implemented. Tables 2-1 and 2-2 address the requirements for the home environment and management of supplies and equipment. If there are any concerns about the home environment, the HHD nurse will perform a home visit to confirm suitability before a patient begins training.

There are basic skills that need to be assessed as part of the screening evaluation. If the patient is unable to meet all physical and psychosocial criteria, then an appropriate support person must be available and interested in performing this role. Necessary skills include ability to read at a fifth grade reading level or higher and ability to memorize skills that they learn. The patient must have sufficient eyesight to read text for written directions. Eyesight and ability to read can be tested by asking a patient to read two short sentences that are typed in a small (10) and large (20) font size. The cloze deletion test is a simple test method to measure comprehension. A Mini-Mental State Exam can be done to assess cognition. Sufficient hearing, so patients can participate

Table 2-1 REQUIREMENTS FOR THE HOME ENVIRONMENT	
Home Environment	
Own or rent home	If renting, need verification that modifications to the home can be made and that there are no restrictions for HHD
Water sources and drains	Municipal: Sufficient water pressure Well water: Testing to ensure adequate water supply Water source within 40 feet of the dialysis treatment area Drain or sink within 40 feet of the dialysis treatment area Septic tank or municipal sewer: Septic tank must accommodate 60 L of fluid per day
Phone	Landline Cell phone only (reliability) Internet phone
Pets	Need to stay out of dialysis treatment area during put on and take off

Table 2-2   MANAGEMENT OF SUPPLIES AND EQUIPMENT
Supplies and Equipment
Sufficient and appropriate (clean and dry) space for supplies
Ability to carry supplies from storage space to dialysis treatment area
Ability to manage supply inventory and order new supplies
Ability to be home to accept supplies
Ability to dispose of supplies properly
Ability to purchase supplies not included with dialysis supplies (paper towels, garbage bags, chair, etc.)
Appropriate space for dialysis machine and water treatment

during training and hear alarms and warnings while dialyzing at home, can be evaluated by determining if patients utilize a hearing device and if they appear to have difficulty hearing during normal conversation. The Ishihara Test for Color Blindness should also be performed.[4] The patient must have sufficient strength and dexterity to lift a bag of dialysate and set up the machine.

Additionally, there should be an assessment of the patient's ability to adhere to the treatment schedule, including the HHD training period, and ability to communicate effectively. If a care partner will be assisting the patient, further assessment should take place to delineate the respective roles of the patient and care partner and to understand the patient to care partner relationship. Assessing for mental illness as well as psychosocial support is also important so that the HHD care team can be more prepared to support the patient once they are on HHD.

To avoid any misunderstandings as training progresses, the screening evaluation meeting needs to include a review of program expectations (Table 2-3). This includes a detailed review of the training process, which can take 4 to 6 weeks and may require scheduled time off from work. Patients should be made aware that their responsibilities include participating fully in training, cannulating the vascular access, maintaining treatment records, drawing labs, ordering supplies, and communicating regularly with the HHD nurse. Requirements for the home environment and managing equipment should also be reviewed again (Tables 2-1 and 2-2). Finally, during the in-person screening evaluation, the team should compile pertinent medical information that may identify medical problems that might make HHD challenging or alert the team to problems that might occur during training or when the patient is dialyzing at home.

Table 2-3   SAMPLE SCREENING EVALUATION MEETING WITH PATIENT TO ADDRESS RESPONSIBILITIES
Patient Responsibilities
Train 4–5 days per week until completed and competent to dialyze at home
Expect possible adjustments to medications and dry weight
Learn to cannulate
Maintain treatment records and submit to facility
Draw monthly labs
Keep emergency items in good working order:
Phone
Flashlight
Emergency kit
Call emergency service and then home facility for emergencies
Attend monthly and as-needed clinic appointments
Notify clinic about changes in living situation

▌ PATIENT TRAINING

Training of the HHD patient can be separated into initial training (before treatments start at home), and follow-up training, which should continue for the duration of time that the patient is performing HHD. The initial training period, which is often 4 to 6 weeks or longer, is fundamental to learning safety and technique of the procedure. However, all HHD patients require consistent, ongoing review of topics as well, which can be either incorporated into the monthly visit or scheduled separately as mandatory retraining sessions. The rationale behind this retraining is that patients may become less strict with technique as they grow more comfortable dialyzing at home and this may potentially increase the risk of complications. Given that a guiding principle of a home dialysis program is "safety first," we are obligated to ensure that patients performing HHD have perfect skills.

Training will differ depending on the dialysis machine the patient elects to use. Currently, there are three HD platforms approved by the FDA for use in the home, though other machines may be available in the near future. The Fresenius 2008K@home and the NxStage System One are both approved for short daily hemodialysis (SDHD) and NHD. The NxStage system does not require a partner. In March 2020, the Tablo Hemodialysis System was approved for use in the home.

Cannulating the vascular access is a key part of HHD training, and for many patients, the most anxiety-provoking aspect. HHD patients use both the rope ladder and buttonhole techniques, and the pros and cons of each option should be discussed with the patient prior to training. If the plan is for buttonholes, the patient, and not the nurse, should create them. As in all HD, vascular access complications are associated with increased morbidity and mortality. Training, and ongoing retraining of self-cannulation, is fundamental for patients to avoid complications. A vascular access nurse-administered checklist can be used, which has been shown to decrease the number of errors over time.[5,6]

The ideal training program should be standardized with a clear ordering of topics. However, the program should have some options and flexibility when it comes to method of teaching and the amount of time that is spent on each topic. Adult learners who are training for HHD can have different educational backgrounds and preferred learning methods. VARK, for instance, is a validated questionnaire that examines different adult learning preferences and categorizes them into visual (V), auditory (A), reading-writing (R), and kinesthetic (K). At a minimum, there should be informal discussion between the training nurse and patient to establish preferred methods of learning so that the nurse can customize and review the material in a way that will be easiest for the patient to learn.[7] Reference materials should have sufficient illustrations/photographs and diagrams available for more visual learners, in addition to text. Training manuals should be provided to the patient for reading and review.

Expectations of the program should be reviewed at the beginning of training, including what the patient can expect from the training nurse and what the center can expect from the patient. Some programs use agreements that are signed and dated. Ideally, one training nurse works daily with the patient for the duration of training to ensure consistency in teaching and allow a comfortable working relationship to form. The training is designed to be completed over a 6-week period, but may take less or more time depending on how easily the patient learns and masters the material, and whether they are also learning to cannulate the vascular access.

The physician should be in regular communication with the training nurse to discuss how training is proceeding and anticipate any barriers to successful completion. Ideally, the physician should see the patient at least once during treatment and document a training visit. The physician is responsible for prescribing the correct dialysis treatment, adjusting medications (e.g., changing intravenous in-center HD medications to oral alternatives), making sure the access is appropriate for use, helping determine best location for buttonhole placement, and verifying that the patient's home is suitable for HHD. The physician also needs to reinforce the importance of communication and teamwork and should underscore the central role of the nursing staff in making sure the patient is performing dialysis safely at home.

A complete procedure checklist is used to ensure that patients can independently perform each task by the end of training. A sample of the type of procedures included in the list is shown in Table 2-4. During training, this procedure checklist is used to document when the task is initially taught, when the patient independently demonstrated the skill for the nurse, and when the patient acknowledged capability to perform the skill independently. There is a subset of skills, which are the minimum requirements for a patient's care partner to be considered a trained helper. These include ability to terminate the treatment if needed, understanding of adverse reactions of medications that are administered at home, recognition of indications for and ability to administer normal saline, as well as knowledge of potential emergencies and adverse events related to the dialysis procedure and vascular access. When a care partner is training with a patient, one strategy that can be used is to first train the patient, and then have the patient train his/her partner. For instance, the patient may attend training alone during week 1, and then in week 2, the partner joins and is taught by the patient. This will allow the nurse to observe how much the patient truly understands, and build confidence for the patient when they successfully train their partner. It also helps define the relationship between the patient and partner regarding responsibility for different aspects of the treatment.

Some patients will dialyze alone without a partner. At least one HHD machine has specific indication for dialysis without a partner; the language for the other home machines is vague and does not forbid dialysis without a partner. In principle, the training process and requirements are the same except that the patient will be responsible for all aspects of their care. They will not have someone to help avoid a mistake during treatment, assist them when they need help, or take over if the patient has a concurrent illness and cannot do their dialysis. Training must be adjusted accordingly, with special attention to addressing possible emergencies. The absence of support can be very taxing and burdensome for some patients. They need to be reminded periodically, even if they are doing well, that respite care is always available. It is much better to identify a problem and intercede early before the patient has a potential crisis at home.

Patients complete a mid-training evaluation, usually after 2 weeks, which serves as a way to review how training is going and encourage open communication between the patient and trainer nurse. At this juncture, it is important to decide if the patient is doing well enough to continue

Table 2-4 SAMPLE OF PROCEDURE CHECKLIST USED FOR HHD TRAINING

Topics Covered During HHD Training with Examples

Infection control
　Appropriate precautions
　Disposal of contaminated waste
　Hand washing technique
Operation of dialysis delivery system
　Understand system alarms
　Machine disinfection procedure
　Machine setup
Hemodialysis procedure
　Verify prescription
　Document treatment data on the flowsheet
　Initiate treatment
　Obtain necessary lab work
　Calculate fluid removal goals
　Monitor during treatment
Vascular access procedures
　Evaluate and examine the access
　Properly cannulate the access
　Use proper technique to tape and secure bloodlines
　Monitor for signs and symptoms of infection or other access complication
Medication: Preparation and administration
　Understand indications and action of medications
　Document medication administration
　Use aseptic technique for administration of medications
　Know indications for use of normal saline during treatment
Risks and complications of hemodialysis
　Respond to medical complications
　　Cramping
　　Nausea/vomiting
　　Chest pain
　　Hypotension
　　Allergic reaction
　　Fever
Technical problems
　Clotting in the bloodlines
　Dialyzer blood leak
　Problems with blood flow
　Emergency termination of treatment
　Hand cranking in event of a power failure

(Continued)

Table 2-4   SAMPLE OF PROCEDURE CHECKLIST USED FOR HHD TRAINING (*CONTINUED*)
Topics Covered During HHD Training with Examples

Laboratory procedures
  Sample collection
  Collection of dialysis adequacy
  Machine water sample
Operation and use of ancillary equipment
  Conductivity meter
  Glucometer if needed
Dialysate bath procedures
  Storage of acid and bicarbonate concentration
  pH testing of dialysate
  Proper cleaning and disinfecting techniques
Water treatment
  Understand process of water treatment
  Testing of water hardness, chlorine/chloramine, water treatment system
  How to document results and report abnormal results

training, identify problems that need correction prior to proceeding, or determine that there are too many serious concerns that preclude further training. During this mid-training evaluation, the patient and nurse discuss whether the patient is appropriately learning proper techniques for performing HHD treatments safely and adequately, and growing comfortable with safety procedures. They also discuss the patient's support system and address whether either party has concerns or anticipates barriers to adherence to treatments. If there are any concerns about a patient successfully completing training and dialyzing at home, these should be identified and discussed—the physician should also participate in such discussions. Sometimes the patient needs a break and does in-center HD for a period (perhaps several weeks), while they reconsider their decision to pursue HHD. Once concerns are addressed and corrected, all parties sign the mid-training evaluation form to document the agreement to complete HHD training.

At the end of training, full competency is reviewed prior to starting treatments at home. The first treatment at home can be very difficult for the patient; therefore, the nurse is present for at least one treatment. During the home visit, the nurse verifies that the home is safe and suitable for HHD treatments and that the setup at home is complete. They help determine the best location and positioning of the machine and help arrange storage of supplies to make the process as efficient as possible. The nurse's presence at the patient's home for the first treatment will help alleviate anxiety and ensure proper technique in the home environment. The nurse may need to help the patient at home for several treatments.

There should always be a nurse available on call for patient questions or emergencies, and patients should be reminded of this regularly. They should always have emergency contact information readily available next to or attached to their machine, in their wallet, and entered into their phone. They are taught that in the event of an emergency such as a power outage or alarms that they cannot quickly correct, it is safer for them to just stop treatment and lose the blood in the extracorporeal dialysis circuit rather than incorrectly perform a function that might put their health in danger.

After a patient has been dialyzing successfully at home, and processes become second nature, there is an increased risk for skipping steps and relaxing technique. This potential concern should be discussed with patients upfront and there should be a plan in place for regular retraining of the patient. Retraining can be scheduled at regular monthly clinic visits, or separately as mandatory retraining sessions. A list of topics which should be included during retraining and suggested frequency of review are provided in Table 2-5.

[For more information, see Chapters 3 and 4.]

▌CARE PARTNERS

Most patients train with a care partner. The role of the care partner can range from serving as a support person with minimal hands-on participation in the treatment, to fully performing all treatment-related tasks. The division of labor between the patient and care partner should be clearly discussed during screening and documented at the beginning of training. Although for many patients the care partner is a family member (spouse, parent, or child), this is not always the case. It is important to understand the patient–care partner dynamic early on and support them both during training. Training for and performing HHD treatments at home can become a source of burden or stress to either party, and discussing and assessing this psychosocial component with the patient and care partner during training is extremely important for their ultimate success on HHD.[8]

Table 2-5 SUGGESTED TOPICS FOR RETRAINING	
HHD Patient Education Retraining Topics	**Frequency**
1. Review emergency procedures at home/disaster planning	4 times/year
2. Review adequacy testing and specimen collection	2 times/year
3. Review home environment (electrical/plumbing), supply ordering, and home inventory	2 times/year
4. Review disinfection/RO procedure, documentation of water and dialysate testing, lab draw technique	2 times/year
5. Review policies for emergency supplies, travel policy	2 times/year
6. Review patient flow sheet records	2 times/year
7. Review fluid balance, volume overload, dehydration, and determining UF goals	2 times/year
8. Review strategies to avoid intradialytic symptoms	2 times/year
9. Review common ESKD medications including for bone mineral and anemia	2 times/year
10. Review daily routine access care, access emergencies	2 times/year
11. Review signs/symptoms of infection and appropriate step to take	2 times/year
12. Review diet, albumin goals	2 times/year
13. Review bone mineral balance and phosphorus binder use and targets	2 times/year
14. Review strategies for managing medications	2 times/year
15. Review treatment options/transplantation status	2 times/year
16. Discuss burden of therapy, resources available, support options	2 times/year
17. Review aseptic technique (masking/hand washing) and disposal of home waste	4 times/year

▍REFERENCES

1. Goovaents T, Jadoul M, Goffin E. Influence of a pre-dialysis education programme (PDEP) on the mode of renal replacement therapy. *Nephrol Dial Transplant.* 2005;20:1842-1847.

2. Robar A, Moran J. The effect of education on patient therapy choice. *Perit Dial Int*. 2007;27(suppl 1):S25.

3. Rioux JP, Cheema H, Bargman JM, Watsin D, Chan CT. Effect of an in-hospital chronic kidney disease education program among patient with unplanned urgent-start dialysis. *Clin J Soc Nephrol*. 2011;6:799-804.

4. Clark JH. The Ishihara test for color blindness. *Am J Physiol Opt*. 1924;5:269-276.

5. Rousseau-Gagnon M, Faratro R, D'Gama C, et al. The use of vascular access audit and infections in home hemodialysis. *Hemodial Int*. 2015;20:298-305.

6. Dhruve M, Faratro R, D'Gama C, et al. The use of nurse-administered vascular access audit in home hemodialysis patients: a quality initiative. *Hemodial Int*. 2019;23:133-138.

7. Auguste BL, Al-Muhaiteeba A, Chan CT. The effect of learning styles on adverse events in home hemodialysis patients. *Clin J Am Soc Nephrol*. 2018;13:782-783.

8. Chan CT, Wallace E, Golper TA, et al. Exploring barriers and potential solutions in home dialysis: an NKF-KDOQI conference outcomes report. *Am J Kidney Dis*. 2019;73(3):363-371.

3 VASCULAR ACCESS FOR HOME HEMODIALYSIS

Anil K. Agarwal, Khaled Y. Boubes, and Nabil F. Haddad

TYPES AND CHOICE OF HOME HEMODIALYSIS VASCULAR ACCESS

Hemodialysis (HD) is the dialysis modality for approximately 63% of all prevalent end-stage kidney disease (ESKD) patients in the United States, with only 2% of all HD patients dialyzing at home as of December 31,

2016.[1] The number of prevalent patients on home therapies (including 7% of patients utilizing peritoneal dialysis [PD]) is difficult to reconcile with the desired goal of 80% of incident patients starting with either home dialysis therapy or transplantation by year 2025 as proclaimed by the American Kidney Health Initiative executive order in July 2019.

HD remains the dialysis modality of choice around the world. It is well known that an arteriovenous fistula (AVF) or an arteriovenous graft (AVG) is superior to a tunneled dialysis catheter (TDC) in terms of outcomes. Despite various initiatives to improve AVF use, approximately 80% of incident patients start HD with a catheter in the United States and nearly 20% of the prevalent patients still use a TDC. Thus, all types of dialysis access, including AVF, AVG, and TDC, will need to be considered for home hemodialysis (HHD) in both incident and prevalent patients.

[For more information, see Chapter 14.]

Characteristics of Vascular Access for Home Hemodialysis

A vascular access that can be cannulated or accessed by the patient (or care partner) with consistency at home is the key to success in enabling the patient to "go home." HHD also presents a unique challenge as, in most instances, the responsibility of the vascular access connection to the dialysis machine is placed upon the patient or a care partner, who is most frequently a family member. Moreover, an access may be used more frequently (four to six times a week compared to only thrice-weekly in in-center HD). Failure to have an easily accessible and stable vascular access is perhaps one of the most significant barriers to HHD initiation and maintenance and can lead to patient and care partner fatigue with subsequent technique failure. Therefore, it is crucial for a successful HHD program to establish an excellent vascular access management program for home.

Access Preparation for Home Hemodialysis

Due to the rather tumultuous and at times chaotic clinical, social, and psychological environment surrounding dialysis initiation, the process of access creation is often poorly organized or deferred. Vascular access management should start before renal replacement therapy (RRT) and a patient, starting on HHD should consider both an arteriovenous (AV) access and a TDC depending upon their ESKD life plan. Establishing a step-wise approach can ensure vessel mapping and scheduling for AV access creation in most cases, although a TDC can remain as a final access for a minority of select individuals. Similarly, in a more stable prevalent patient, it is optimal to proceed with AV access creation, although it should not delay the transition to home. Once an access is obtained, the patient or the care partner should be trained for cannulation as soon as possible.

ACCESS CANNULATION FOR HOME HEMODIALYSIS

Cannulation of an AV access is perhaps the most essential step in transitioning a patient to HHD. Faulty cannulation can cause excessive pain, failure to cannulate, infiltration, bleeding, and trauma leading to aneurysm formation. Incorrect technique also increases the risk of access thrombosis and loss of patency.

Needle Gauge

In general, cannulation should start with small gauge needles (17 gauge) to minimize vessel injury, infiltration, and hematoma formation. The blood flow rate (mL/min) varies according to the needle gauge, being <300 mL/min for 17 gauge, 300 to 350 mL/min for 16 gauge, 350 to 400 mL/min for 15 gauge, and >450 mL/min for 14-gauge needles. However, it is important to remember that most patients on HHD will not require the highest blood flow rates and it is preferable to use the smallest possible needle gauge needed to achieve adequacy.

Cannulation Techniques

The two most common cannulation techniques used for AVF cannulation are a rotating site technique, known as the "rope-ladder" technique, and a constant site technique, known as the "buttonhole" technique. It is to be noted that "area" cannulation of an AVF, meaning repeated cannulations within the same adjacent area of an AVF close together, will eventually weaken the vein wall resulting in aneurysm formation and must be avoided.

Rope-ladder cannulation

Site rotation (or rope-ladder technique) is considered the more desirable technique for most patients with a reasonable length of AVF available for cannulation. In this method, the cannulation site is rotated, using a sharp needle each time. This technique allows healing of previous sites while other sites are used, and reduces the likelihood of aneurysm formation.

Buttonhole cannulation

Buttonhole cannulation of AVF requires creation of well-formed "button-holes" by using a constant site, angle, depth, and direction of needle for cannulation. Typically, repeated cannulation with sharp needles (usually 8 to 10 times) of the site is required to create a cannulation track. Once the track is mature, blunt needles can be used to access the AVF after carefully removing the overlying scab (Figure 3-1A and B). Polycarbonate peg (e.g., BioHole Plug, Supercath) can be used to create a buttonhole, and their dull versions are used later to cannulate for performance of HD.[2] It is recommended that a single operator should create a buttonhole using a constant angle, position of the arm, and tourniquet placement with each cannulation.[3] Although the angle of needle entry will vary with the site, depth, and the anatomy of the AVF in every patient, it should remain constant in a particular patient at each cannulation (Figure 3-2). A second pair of buttonholes can be created for alternating use of buttonholes; however, if unused, the buttonhole track may quickly close.[4]

Prior to cannulation of a buttonhole for HD, the overlying scab needs to be removed and every program must develop a protocol for proper removal of scab. This protocol may involve prolonged soaking of the

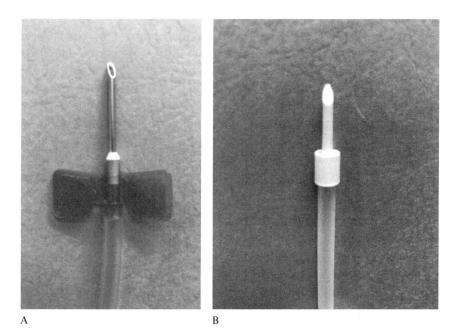

A   B

Figure 3-1 • Sharp (A) and blunt dialysis needles (B).

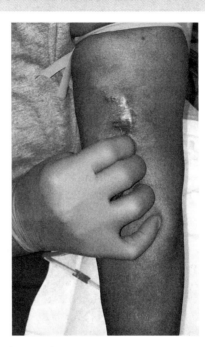

Figure 3-2 • Buttonhole cannulation.

buttonhole and gentle removal of scab without using a sharp needle, or a sterile sharp needle may also be used to remove the scab. The needle that is used to remove scab must never be used for cannulation of the buttonhole, or the skin flora will be introduced into the blood stream increasing the risk of bacteremia.

Buttonhole cannulation has many disadvantages. In many cases, a tract may fail to develop, which may be related to inconsistent technique. At times, the patient may need sharp needle cannulation at a different site if there is difficulty in buttonhole cannulation or when unfamiliar or inexperienced operators do the cannulation. A buttonhole may also need to be recreated if the track moves (due to scarring) or becomes infected. AVF stenosis has been noted at the site of buttonholes, although this has not been investigated in prospective studies.

Infection is the single biggest risk associated with buttonhole cannulation as demonstrated in both observational and randomized controlled studies, although results have varied between studies. An increased risk of bacteremia and localized signs of infection were noted in a randomized study.[5] In a retrospective analysis of infectious complications, the bacteremia rate was noted to be 0.073 per 1000 AVF days for buttonhole, compared to none for rope-ladder.[6] A systematic review showed an approximately three times higher risk of infection with buttonhole as well as increased staff support requirements and no reduction in surgical AVF interventions compared with rope-ladder technique.[7] Based on these findings, it has been suggested by some authors that the use of buttonhole cannulation should be abandoned.

However, buttonhole cannulation provides an important method of facilitating cannulation in HHD and other selected patients if meticulous technique can be followed. Multiple small observational studies have advocated the use of buttonhole technique. There was decreased hematoma and aneurysm formation in prevalent HD patients using buttonholes.[8] A prospective observational study in South Korea showed improved hemostasis time, cannulation pain, and nursing stress without a change in vascular access blood flow rate and dialysis adequacy in HD patients using buttonhole cannulation.[4] In the study of BioHole-assisted buttonhole creation, AVF survival was better when using buttonhole cannulation as compared to rope-ladder cannulation.[2] The buttonhole technique was also noted to significantly decrease the need for access interventions and reduce existing aneurysm enlargement without an increase in infection rates or prolonged bleeding times.

Thus, selection of a cannulation technique requires consideration of individual patient needs and feasibility without immediately accepting or rejecting a technique. Both rope-ladder and buttonhole techniques, when used carefully using a constant protocol, have the potential to support long-term HHD without complications.

[For more information, see Chapters 7 and 8.]

Selection of cannulation technique

Buttonhole cannulation is not suitable for every patient. Ideally, buttonholes are helpful to those with a short AVF with limited area available for cannulation, so that rotation of sites is not feasible. This may occur when the majority of the AVF is either deep, tortuous, or aneurysmal. Sometimes, the patient desiring to go home is simply unable to self-cannulate using rope-ladder technique even though multiple cannulation sites are possible. Patients may also prefer buttonhole cannulation due to pain intolerance or fear of needles. However, a patient with poor vision or hand tremors may not be able to follow the exact cannulation technique. Patients with an indwelling prosthesis are at risk of infection from potential bacteremia and are not considered good candidates for buttonhole cannulation.[3]

Cannulation of arteriovenous graft for home hemodialysis

Cannulation of an AVG is usually easier than cannulation of an AVF. Standard sharp needles or the needles with cannula (angiocatheters) can be used. An important reminder for AVG cannulation is that an AVG should only be cannulated with rotating site technique, not buttonhole, because a constant track in an AVG cannot heal and a buttonhole has a higher likelihood of bleeding and pseudoaneurysm formation, eventually leading to the serious complications of infection and bleeding.

SELF-CANNULATION AT HOME: BARRIERS AND COMPLICATIONS

A small and deep access, especially on the dominant extremity, can be especially challenging to self-cannulate. Lack of experience and inadequate training can make cannulation impossible. Trypanophobia (fear of needles) and hemophobia (fear of blood) are psychological barriers, which can be alleviated with proper training, education, and support. Patients and care partners perceive that HHD offers the opportunity to thrive—it improves freedom, flexibility, and well-being, and strengthens relationships.[9] However, anxiety and fear of starting a very involved and daunting HHD treatment in isolation from medical and social support can be overwhelming. Care partner fatigue is common and requires staff support. Occasionally, the patients may require respite in-center HD during a period of high stress at home.

Difficult and faulty cannulation can lead to multiple complications. If hygienic measures and sterile technique are not strictly followed, infectious complications may result. Frequent access infiltrations associated with frequent cannulation can severely damage an AVF/AVG and have the potential to negatively impact primary or secondary patency of the access.

Promoting Self-Cannulation

Patients and care partners are especially concerned about the process of dialyzing at home due to the fear of self-cannulation, fear of needles, and bleeding complications. Identification of patient barriers followed by methods to navigate those barriers are required.[10] Assessment and mapping of access by the staff and patient together may help in cannulation. A patient's fear may be eased by support from staff, hand holding, warm compresses, and local anesthetics. Various exposure therapy, hypnotherapy, relaxation techniques, and medications may also help to alleviate anxiety.

Single Needle Cannulation

A dual lumen single needle may have some advantages for frequent access cannulation. By reducing the number of cannulation sites and likelihood of damage, it has the potential to increase access survival.[11] It may also increase safety by reducing accidental needle dislodgements. However, it may reduce dose of dialysis by decreasing effective dialysis time and increasing the degree of access recirculation, depending upon the needle design. Additional training for cannulation is required with single needle due to the increased risk of infiltration if not fully inserted. Single needles for HD are limited in availability at this time, although newer needles are in development.

MONITORING AND SURVEILLANCE OF VASCULAR ACCESS AFTER MATURATION

The monitoring of a vascular access includes the examination and evaluation of the access to detect physical signs suggesting pathology. If detected, interventions can be planned to prevent access complications. Monitoring is easily done at home. An access examination should be done before every cannulation (at least weekly), starting with the first treatment. It is important to note changes in skin color, circulation, and integrity compared to the other extremity. The development of swelling and erythema may signify the presence of cellulitis or abscess (Figure 3-3). The patient should

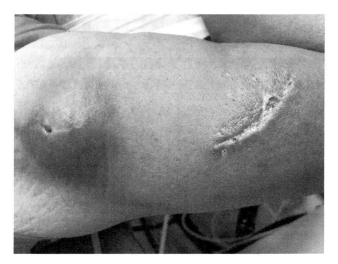

Figure 3-3 • An abscess complicating a buttonhole cannulation site.

look for the presence of edema, drainage, and aneurysms and listen with a stethoscope for any changes in the bruit. A well-functioning AVF has a continuous machine-like bruit as compared to a stenotic fistula, which has a discontinuous, pulse-like, "systolic" bruit that can be high-pitched, musical, or loud. Clues to access dysfunction should be recognized early for timely intervention (Table 3-1).

Surveillance of a vascular access is comprised of periodic evaluation by tests requiring special instruments to detect dysfunction. These tests include measurement of access flow, intra-access pressure and resistance, and Doppler duplex ultrasound imaging. These methods are not readily available at home but can be requested if necessary.

┃ PREVENTION OF ARTERIOVENOUS ACCESS
┃ INFECTION IN HOME HEMODIALYSIS

A cannulation protocol to prevent infection should be used and taught to the patients during training. Important components of the protocol should include the following:

- Strict aseptic technique with gloves and masks
- Disinfectant use for site cleansing prior to cannulation
- Topical antimicrobial prophylaxis of cannulation sites after dialysis
- *Staphylococcus aureus* nasal carriage screening and mupirocin treatment as needed
- Routine audit of patient cannulation technique done quarterly at clinic visit

Table 3-1   CLUES TO PRESENCE OF ACCESS DYSFUNCTION
Difficult cannulation
High arterial or venous pressures
Poor dialysis adequacy
Prolonged bleeding after dialysis
Swelling of extremity
Aneurysm formation or enlargement of access

TUNNELED DIALYSIS CATHETERS FOR HOME HEMODIALYSIS

Many patients, especially incident dialysis patients, will need to use a TDC both for initiation of HHD, and then again during periods of AV access complications for continuation of HD. An internal jugular vein is the preferred site for a TDC. Subclavian vein cannulation should be avoided due to a high incidence of central vein stenosis. While not preferred, a catheter may be a suitable permanent access in selected patients.

Infection, thrombosis, and central vein stenosis are common complications of TDC. Strict aseptic technique and use of a checklist (e.g., use of gloves, masks, and soaking of catheter hubs with antimicrobial solution, etc.) are important to avoid TDC infection. A strict protocol that includes use of appropriate locking solution (e.g., heparin, citrate) after HD is essential. Tissue plasminogen activator is effective in decreasing infection and thrombosis and can be used as a lock solution in selected cases. Dressing with a gauze or a non occlusive transparent dressing and use of topical antimicrobial prophylaxis at the exit site (e.g., polysporin, mupirocin, medi-honey, or povidone-iodine) are recommended. Showers should be avoided, unless a strict protocol is used to cover the TDC. Swimming is also prohibited with a TDC.

Catheter-related infections should be promptly recognized. Exit site infections should be treated with topical antibiotics. Tunnel infections require catheter removal and replacement at a different site. Bacteremia and metastatic infections must be treated with catheter removal, prolonged systemic antibiotics, and possibly antibiotic locks.

A catheter thrombosis management protocol should also be established for HHD. Methods to treat thrombosis include saline forced flush and tissue plasminogen activator instillation. Catheter exchange with treatment of fibrin sheath (if present) may be needed if other measures fail. Central vein stenosis is a serious complication of TDC and can be prevented by avoidance of TDC if AV access can be achieved. Mechanical damage of TDC (e.g., kinked or damaged port) requires repair or exchange with a new catheter.

Closed catheter connector devices have recently emerged as an important method of avoiding infection (Tego connectors, Curos Caps). These devices can also reduce risk of bleeding and air embolism in HHD.

BLEEDING COMPLICATIONS OF VASCULAR ACCESS IN HOME HEMODIALYSIS

Hemorrhage of varying severity has been reported in HHD but is relatively rare. Hemorrhage usually occurs as a result of needle dislodgement or misthreading of the arterial tubing to the dialyzer and can result in exsanguination, which is extremely rare. A rapidly enlarging aneurysm with thin or necrotic skin should be repaired promptly to avoid hemorrhage from the access (Figure 3-4). Proper needle taping technique involves placing an initial strip of tape over the needle, crisscrossing another strip of tape, and covering with yet another strip. Additionally, the tubing is taped near the shoulder to avoid accidental needle dislodgement. Water or enuresis alarms can be strategically placed under the dialysis machine, dialyzer, as well as under the access arm to quickly detect blood loss.

[For more information, see Chapter 8.]

ANTICOAGULATION FOR HOME HEMODIALYSIS VASCULAR ACCESS

There are no special protocols for anticoagulation for HHD and usual clinic protocols should be followed. Generally, heparin bolus is used and infusion is avoided. No meaningful benefit of antiplatelet therapy has been noted in studies of dialysis vascular access and these therapies are not recommended unless needed for another reason.

[For more information, see Chapter 8.]

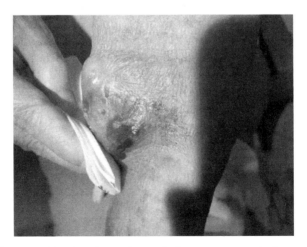

Figure 3-4 • Active bleeding from a buttonhole aneurysm site indicating potentially imminent rupture.

EXPERIENCE IN USING VASCULAR ACCESS FOR HOME HEMODIALYSIS

Vascular access outcomes have been studied in the setting of HHD, more frequent HD, and nocturnal hemodialysis (NHD). Reports of successful use of AVF for HHD date back to the 1960s.[12] Several studies comparing different types of vascular access in the HHD population are available but most are retrospective observational studies and the number of randomized controlled trials is small. In a large cohort of patients ($N = 2543$), outcomes were analyzed according to the type of vascular access at the start of HHD.[13] Catheter use was associated with a higher risk of mortality and hospitalization, but not with transfer to in-center HD. Another observational study showed 37% reduction in the mortality risk with AV access when compared with TDC, although technique survival was not affected.[14] A small study from the United Kingdom showed primary and secondary patency of AV access at 1 year as 78% and 100%, respectively.[15] In a study of 286 HD patients in Australia, increased frequency and/or duration of dialysis was associated with excellent survival rates.[16] Most adverse events were related to vascular access complications, mainly infection. The Australia and New Zealand registry noted the highest mortality among in-center HD with TDC group and lowest in the HHD with AV access group.[17] Further, HHD with AV access had better mortality than in-center HD with AV access.

Vascular access–related infections have also been examined in HHD. A retrospective study from Canada ($N = 187$) noted a bacteremia rate as high as 1.12 episodes per 1000 patient days for the TDC group compared to only 0.25 episodes per 1000 patient days in the AV access group.[18] Infections were due to gram-positive bacteria in 74.6% of the episodes and gram-negative bacteria in 24.7%, with one case of a fungal infection. Coagulase negative *Staphylococcus* (51.4%) were the most common organisms isolated followed by *Staphylococcus aureus* (20.3%). An observational study utilized the US Renal Data System (USRDS) to examine complications in 3480 HHD patients and 17,400 thrice-weekly in-center HD patients.[19] In the intention-to-treat analysis, HHD patients, compared to in-center HD cohorts, had similar risk of all-cause hospital admissions but higher risk of admission for vascular access infections.

VASCULAR ACCESS OUTCOMES IN MORE FREQUENT HEMODIALYSIS

Early studies of frequent HD showed variable results and were limited by sample size and design characteristics. A systematic review of 12 studies found that patients on daily HD, as compared to those on thrice-weekly HD, had no apparent increase in vascular access complications and perhaps even better outcomes for vascular access prognosis.[20] Subsequently, in the Frequent Hemodialysis Network (FHN) Trial (a randomized trial of 120 patients on conventional hemodialysis [CHD] of three times per week and 125 patients on more frequent HD of six times per week) found that more frequent HD was associated with more vascular access interventions (95 interventions in the more frequent HD group and 65 in the CHD group).[21] At least one procedure was required in 47% of more frequent HD cohort but only in 29% in the thrice-weekly HD group. In the CHD group, the percentage of interventions in AVF, AVG, and TDC was 48%, 38%, and 14%, respectively, while in the more frequent HD group this percentage for AVF, AVG, and TDC was 51%, 32%, and 17%, respectively.

The FHN Nocturnal Trial (a randomized trial of 42 patients on thrice-weekly CHD and 45 patients on six times per week home NHD) showed patients on nocturnal HHD had a trend toward higher vascular access complications.[22] There were a total of 34 vascular access events (17 failures and 17 access interventions) in the NHD group versus 21 events (13 failures and 8 access procedures) in the CHD group. The percentage of vascular access events in the NHD group was 50% in AVF, 6% in AVG, and 44% in TDC, while in the CHD cohort it was 19% in AVF, 24% in AVG, and 57% in TDC. Vascular access procedure or failure occurred in 51% of NHD patients as compared to 36% CHD patients with a hazard ratio for time to first access event of 1.88 ($P = 0.06$).

Another 4-year prospective observational study of six versus three times per week HD recorded total access procedures (fistulagram, thrombectomy, and access revision). There were 543.2 procedures per 1000 person-years in CHD versus 400.8 procedures per 1000 person-years in the more frequent HD group. There was no difference in time to first access revision between the more frequent HD and the CHD groups. Consequently, this study concluded that more frequent HD was not associated with increased access complications or increased access failure rates.[23]

More recently, overall complications of vascular access were examined with more frequent HD in two separate randomized controlled trials. A total of 198 patients with AVF or AVG and 47 patients with TDC received 6 days per week of in-center HD versus 3 days per week of CHD; and 87 patients received 6 nights per week of home NHD or 3 days per week of HHD for 12 months.[24] More total AV access procedures were needed in more frequent HD (both home and in-center) patients compared to patients on less frequent CHD; 55% of all interventions involved thrombectomies and surgical revisions. There were 33 repairs and 15 losses in the more frequent HD group as compared to 17 repairs, 11 losses, and 1 hospitalization in the CHD group. The hazard ratio for time to first access repair, loss, or access-related hospitalization was 1.9 in patients with AVF or AVG in the more frequent HD cohort as compared to the CHD group, while it was 2.7 in those with a TDC. The overall risk for a first access event was 76% higher with more frequent HD than with CHD (hazard ratio 1.76) with no difference in loss of AV access between groups.

A meta-analysis of 15 studies analyzing vascular access outcomes included 1540 access-years for more frequent HD and 2284 access-years for CHD.[25] There were higher vascular access event rates in the more frequent HD group, as compared to the CHD group (difference of 6.7 events per 100 patient-years). AVG and TDC had higher event rates when compared to AVF. Overall, there was a higher number of vascular access complications in patients undergoing more frequent HD as compared to CHD.

[For more information, see Chapter 7.]

❚ SUMMARY

Vascular access stability is essential for performance of safe and effective HHD. Almost any type of access can be used for HHD and the choice of access should be individualized. The cannulation technique should be carefully selected and sterile precautions taught and audited periodically. Buttonhole cannulation can be used, but has a higher risk of infection unless a strict aseptic protocol is followed. A protocol-based approach for creation, maintenance, and troubleshooting of vascular access is more likely to enable success in HHD.

❚ REFERENCES

1. United States Renal Data System. 2019 USRDS annual data report: epidemiology of kidney disease in the United States. National Institutes of Health, National Institute of Diabetes and Digestive and Kidney Diseases, Bethesda, MD; 2019.
2. Vaux E, King J, Lloyd S, et al. Effect of buttonhole cannulation with a polycarbonate PEG on in-center hemodialysis fistula outcomes: a randomized controlled trial. *Am J Kidney Dis*. 2013;62(1):81-88.
3. Faratro R, Jeffries J, Nesrallah GE, MacRae JM. The care and keeping of vascular access for home hemodialysis patients. *Hemodial Int*. 2015;19(suppl 1):S80-S92.
4. Kim MK, Kim HS. Clinical effects of buttonhole cannulation method on hemodialysis patients. *Hemodial Int*. 2013;17(2):294-299.

5. MacRae JM, Ahmed SB, Atkar R, Hemmelgarn BR. A randomized trial comparing buttonhole with rope ladder needling in conventional hemodialysis patients. *Clin J Am Soc Nephrol.* 2012;7(10):1632-1638.

6. O'Brien FJ, Kok HK, O'Kane C, et al. Arterio-venous fistula buttonhole cannulation technique: a retrospective analysis of infectious complications. *Clin Kidney J.* 2012;5(6):526-529.

7. Muir CA, Kotwal SS, Hawley CM, et al. Buttonhole cannulation and clinical outcomes in a home hemodialysis cohort and systematic review. *Clin J Am Soc Nephrol.* 2014;9(1):110-119.

8. van Loon MM, Goovaerts T, Kessels AG, van der Sande FM, Tordoir JH. Buttonhole needling of haemodialysis arteriovenous fistulae results in less complications and interventions compared to the rope-ladder technique. *Nephrol Dial Transplant.* 2010;25(1):225-230.

9. Walker RC, Hanson CS, Palmer SC, et al. Patient and caregiver perspectives on home hemodialysis: a systematic review. *Am J Kidney Dis.* 2015;65(3):451-463.

10. Ward FL, Faratro R, McQuillan RF. Self-cannulation of the vascular access in home hemodialysis: overcoming patient-level barriers. *Semin Dial.* 2018;31(5):449-454.

11. Perl J, Chan CT. Home hemodialysis, daily hemodialysis, and nocturnal hemodialysis: core curriculum 2009. *Am J Kidney Dis.* 2009;54(6):1171-1184.

12. Shaldon S, McKay S. Use of internal arteriovenous fistula in home haemodialysis. *Br Med J.* 1968;4(5632):671-673.

13. Rivara MB, Soohoo M, Streja E, et al. Association of vascular access type with mortality, hospitalization, and transfer to in-center hemodialysis in patients undergoing home hemodialysis. *Clin J Am Soc Nephrol.* 2016;11(2):298-307.

14. Perl J, Nessim SJ, Moist LM, et al. Vascular access type and patient and technique survival in home hemodialysis patients: the Canadian Organ Replacement Register. *Am J Kidney Dis.* 2016;67(2):251-259.

15. Al Shakarchi J, Day C, Inston N. Vascular access for home haemodialysis. *J Vasc Access.* 2018;19(6):593-595.

16. Jun M, Jardine MJ, Gray N, et al. Outcomes of extended-hours hemodialysis performed predominantly at home. *Am J Kidney Dis.* 2013;61(2):247-253.

17. Kasza J, Wolfe R, McDonald SP, Marshall MR, Polkinghorne KR. Dialysis modality, vascular access and mortality in end-stage kidney disease: a bi-national registry-based cohort study. *Nephrology.* 2016;21(10):878-886.

18. Hayes WN, Tennankore K, Battistella M, Chan CT. Vascular access-related infection in nocturnal home hemodialysis. *Hemodial Int.* 2014;18(2):481-487.

19. Weinhandl ED, Nieman KM, Gilbertson DT, Collins AJ. Hospitalization in daily home hemodialysis and matched thrice-weekly in-center hemodialysis patients. *Am J Kidney Dis.* 2015;65(1):98-108.

20. Shurraw S, Zimmerman D. Vascular access complications in daily dialysis: a systematic review of the literature. *Minerva Urol Nefrol.* 2005;57(3):151-163.

21. Group FHNT, Chertow GM, Levin NW, et al. In-center hemodialysis six times per week versus three times per week. *N Engl J Med.* 2010;363(24):2287-2300.

22. Rocco MV, Lockridge RS Jr, Beck GJ, et al. The effects of frequent nocturnal home hemodialysis: the Frequent Hemodialysis Network Nocturnal Trial. *Kidney Int*. 2011;80(10):1080-1091.

23. Achinger SG, Ikizler TA, Bian A, Shintani A, Ayus JC. Long-term effects of daily hemodialysis on vascular access outcomes: a prospective controlled study. *Hemodial Int*. 2013;17(2):208-215.

24. Suri RS, Larive B, Sherer S, et al. Risk of vascular access complications with frequent hemodialysis. *J Am Soc Nephrol*. 2013;24(3):498-505.

25. Cornelis T, Usvyat LA, Tordoir JH, et al. Vascular access vulnerability in intensive hemodialysis: a significant Achilles' heel? *Blood Purif*. 2014;37(3):222-228.

4 PRESCRIBING HOME HEMODIALYSIS

Michael A. Kraus and Michelle Carver

Dialysis has primarily been dominated by the conventional three times per week schedule. In the thrice-weekly world, dialysis prescriptions have been based mostly on achieving urea adequacy and managing the symptoms and morbidity associated with dialysis using medications, and expecting the patient to live with some symptoms. However, over the past several years, an interest in expanding home dialysis, specifically home hemodialysis (HHD), has been a focus of dialysis clinicians across the United States. This drive may be attributed to the following factors: growth of peritoneal dialysis (PD) stemming from changes in the payment system, modernization of technology that has decreased the burden of HHD, increasing interest in person-centered care, and increased awareness of the potential benefits of home therapies. This interest has not been missed by the US government, which has actively encouraged the expansion of home dialysis and transplantation through policy reform.

Indeed, HHD provides the opportunity for suitable patients to achieve more frequent dialysis with less burden and greater freedom to travel. Thus, the proper prescription for HHD can allow exploration of "optimal" versus "adequate" dialysis. The optimal dialysis prescription not only provides adequate dialysis but also provides improved volume and blood pressure control, decreasing the medication burden and symptoms associated with end-stage kidney disease (ESKD). Optimal dialysis, as opposed to adequate dialysis, must address sodium and water as the major dialyzable toxins, followed by phosphorus and middle molecular toxins, while maintaining the conventionally held urea adequacy targets. Using currently available technologies, dialysis can be optimized to improve morbidity and possibly even survival, hopefully increasing access to kidney transplant as well.

Dialysis populations across the world continue to increase, but growth in the United States has recently slowed. This growth primarily has been attributed to improved ESKD survival. Nevertheless, mortality rates remain much higher than in the age-matched US population.[1] In fact, this improving survival has flattened out over the last 4 years without further improvement.[2] Conventional three times a week dialysis fails to adequately address high cardiovascular morbidity and mortality, decreased quality-of-life (QOL) measures, high pill burden, and intolerability of conventional dialysis treatments.

HHD provides an opportunity to prescribe more frequent dialysis regimens that may improve overall survival and QOL for ESKD patients. Increasing adoption of HHD requires addressing barriers for both patients and clinicians. Improving modality education and ensuring patients understand all of their dialysis options and the benefits of each is an important initiative in growing home therapies. Lack of healthcare provider exposure to and education about HHD therapy perpetuates lack of familiarity and therefore creates a hesitancy to refer patients. The goal of this chapter is to review dosing and prescription management practices of HHD.

[For more information, see Chapter 14.]

▌BENEFITS OF HOME HEMODIALYSIS

In the past decade, there has been an increase in both observational and randomized controlled data regarding HHD therapy. Survival advantages have been documented in both frequent short daily hemodialysis (SDHD) and nocturnal hemodialysis (NHD).[3] HHD has also been shown to improve blood pressure and volume control, reverse left ventricular hypertrophy (LVH), reduce serum phosphorus levels and pill burden, and increase both mental and physical QOL health scores.[4–7]

[For more information, see Chapter 7.]

▌ DETERMINING PRESCRIPTION OPTIONS

Currently, there are several different approaches to prescribing HHD. The three most common therapy options in the United States are conventional, more frequent daily, and nocturnal therapy. Conventional HHD is typically done on a thrice-weekly treatment schedule with an average of 3.5 to 4 hours per treatment. The clinical benefits of three times a week dialysis at home are similar to those seen with in-center three times a week dialysis schedules. Lifestyle benefits can be seen as treatments occur in the patient's own home allowing patients to create a treatment schedule that suits their lifestyle. Longer duration treatments, such as NHD, have shown observational improvements in mortality. More frequent HHD is defined as four or more treatments per week, with dialysis sessions lasting 2.5 to 3.5 hours per treatment depending on frequency. One of the biggest advantages of a more frequent treatment schedule is mitigating the 2-day treatment gap. The 2-day gap is the 2 days patients go without treatment on conventional three times a week dialysis. Eliminating this gap shows mortality drops by 45% on Monday and Tuesday when more frequent HHD is used versus thrice-weekly in-center hemodialysis (HD).

More frequent HD can also be done with extended treatments of 5.5 hours or greater in duration. Typically, these treatments are done at night while the patient sleeps, with the treatment time being customized to fit the patient's typical sleep schedule. The benefits of longer, more frequent treatments include all the benefits associated with shorter daily treatment schedules but have the added benefits of increased phosphorus clearance, improved sleep and obstructive sleep apnea, and reduced post-dialysis recovery time.[8] Patients who do NHD should also be educated to use additional safety devices during treatment including a vascular access leak detector.

[For more information, see Chapters 7 and 10.]

▌ PRESCRIBING PATIENT-CENTERED THERAPY OPTIONS

When considering which home therapy option is best for the patient, it is important to consider the treatment frequency that will best meet the patient's clinical needs while still accommodating the patient and family's lifestyle. The care team should have a conversation with the patient to educate them on the clinical benefits of each modality. There should be a discussion to assess the patient's goals for home therapy and to ensure that the proposed treatment schedule can be carried out successfully at home. Prior to initiating therapy, a thorough psychosocial evaluation and medical evaluation are necessary to not only establish appropriateness of home therapies but, more importantly, determine optimal therapy options and evaluate teaching and support needed for successful training, initiation, and retention on therapy.

There are two types of dialysis machines used for HHD—conventional dialysis systems adapted for home use and dialysis systems designed specifically for home use. The key difference between these systems is the dialysate flow rate and total dialysate volume. Conventional dialysis machine use dialysate flow rates of 300 to 800 mL/min, whereas dialysate flow rates for home dialysis machines are much lower, typically ranging from 50 to 250 mL/min (or 25% to 50% of blood flow rates).

The overall prescription for HHD can be broken down to three main components:

1. Frequency—driven by clinical indications
2. Weekly or per session time on dialysis—driven by residual renal function (RRF), ultrafiltration (UF) needs, and, in the setting of low-flow dialysate, desired saturation of dialysate
3. Dialysate volume, rate, and composition

[For more information, see Chapter 2.]

Frequency

HHD allows for scheduling dialysis of virtually any frequency. Frequency is the starting decision point for the dialysis prescription. This varies from less than 3 days per week in incremental dialysis, to conventional thrice-weekly, up to daily. The choice of frequency is up to physician discretion but should be based on clinical needs balanced with social needs of the patient and potential care partners.

Incremental dialysis is gaining more recent attention, but it is not well studied. Data collected thus far is limited to patients with preserved glomerular filtration rate (GFR), urine output, low UF rate requirements, and normotensive patients with normal phosphorus and potassium.[9,10] Hence, its overall usefulness in ESKD care remains low and unknown.

Thrice-weekly dialysis can be prescribed with conventional or low-volume dialysate devices. Some studies have shown equivalent survival advantages to more frequent dialysis, but this might be due to selection bias rather than therapy.[11] It is hard to envision that thrice-weekly dialysis at home has significant physiologic benefits over in-center HD, although there may certainly be social and emotional benefits to dialyzing in the home setting versus in a center.

Alternate day or four times a week dialysis offers the ability to eliminate the 2-day gap on thrice-weekly, which has been associated with increased cardiovascular hospitalization and death.[12] If total time is increased above 12 hours weekly, UF rate may decrease as well. The potential cardiovascular and symptom benefits of the therapy have not been studied.

Most of the benefits of more frequent dialysis, either NHD or SDHD, have been studied in 5 to 6 days per week regimens. With 5 to 6 days per week of dialysis, blood pressure is improved with decreased antihypertensive medications, LVH is reversed, cardiovascular-related hospitalizations are reduced, postdialysis fatigue is reduced, hypotension is decreased, and there is evidence to support better mortality.[4] Therefore, for patients with LVH, volume overload, poorly controlled hypertension (HTN), significant dialysis-related symptoms, postdialysis fatigue, pregnancy, uncontrolled hyperphosphatemia, uncontrolled hyperkalemia, or persistent elevated UF rate, a dialysis frequency of 5 to 6 days per week has the best medical evidence for improvement. For a desired phosphorus control without binders, NHD five nights per week has the best results.[13]

[For more information, see Chapters 7, 9, and 10.]

Time per Week

Studies have shown that longer weekly time on treatment is associated with higher survival rates.[14] A minimum of 12 hours a week of dialysis is recommended. Fifteen hours per week will minimize UF rates and ensure saturation with low-volume dialysate devices. Given the flexibility of scheduling treatments at home, one should consider starting with longer treatment time and decreasing time once the patient has stabilized. The patient's UF requirements will also assist in determining the total weekly hours of dialysis needed. As mentioned previously, treatment frequency is most appropriately determined by evaluating the patient's clinical and lifestyle needs. As with hours of dialysis per week, starting with more frequent dialysis treatments and adjusting as medical needs change assists in setting realistic treatment expectations from the start for patients.

Ultrafiltration Rates

An additional consideration is determining UF rates that are safe for dialysis patients. Physiologically, volume overload results in tissue edema, impaired oxygen and metabolite diffusion, distorted tissue architecture, obstruction of capillary blood flow and lymphatic drainage, and disturbed cell-cell interactions. This may ultimately lead to progressive organ dysfunction. Excess fluid or hypervolemia is the most common cause of HTN and LVH and leads to cardiac disease in patients on HD. Volume overload is a major reason for the risk of cardiovascular disease (CVD) in patients with chronic kidney disease (CKD) stage G5, and incidence of volume overload is far greater than in the general population. High UF rates are associated with increased mortality.[15] An evaluation of data from the Hemodialysis Study, an almost-7-year randomized clinical trial of 1846 patients receiving three times per week chronic dialysis compared UF rate in the lowest group (up to 10 mL/kg/h) to rates in the highest (over 13 mL/kg/h).[16] The highest UF rates were associated with increased all-cause and cardiovascular-related mortality. Rapid fluid removal and intradialytic hypotension (IDH) due to high UF rates during dialysis result in recurrent end-organ injury. Recurrent episodes of ischemia in the heart persist even after the return of normal myocardial blood flow, a phenomenon known as myocardial stunning. Myocardial stunning leads to damaged heart muscle and the development of dilated cardiomyopathy. UF rates at or below 8 mL/kg/h suggest lower mortality risk. Longer treatment times, such as with nocturnal therapy, allow for even slower removal rates.

The total dialysis time per week based on UF rates can be determined by the following:

- Weekly UF requirements (in mL)/EDW (kg) = Weight-based UF desired (mL/kg), where UF is ultrafiltration and EDW is the estimated dry weight
- Weight-based UF desired (mL/kg)/Desired UF rate (mL/kg/h) = Hours of dialysis weekly
- Hours of dialysis weekly/treatment frequency = Hours per session required

For example, an 80-kg male on dialysis 5 days per week, with desired UF of 1250 mL daily would have a weight-based desired UF of 8750 mL/80 kg or 109.4 mL/kg. The hours per week of dialysis with a desired UF rate of 8 mL/kg/h would be 109.4 mL/kg/8 mL/kg/h or 13.7 hours of dialysis weekly.

[For more information, see Chapters 7 and 9.]

▌DIALYSATE FLOW RATES

Generating large volumes of high-quality dialysate can be challenging in the home environment. Efficient use of dialysate fluid is essential to

Table 4-1   DIALYSATE VOLUME PER TREATMENT—MALES

Weight	6×/Week	5×/Week	4×/Week	3.5/Week (EOD)
<60 kg	20 L	20 L	25 L	30 L
61–80 kg	20 L	25 L	40 L	50 L
81–100 kg	25 L	30 L	50 L	60 L
101–120 kg	30 L	40 L	50 L	
121–140 kg	30 L	50 L	60 L	

EOD, every other day.

Table 4-2   DIALYSATE VOLUME PER TREATMENT—FEMALES

Weight	6×/Week	5×/Week	4×/Week	3.5/Week (EOD)
<60 kg	20 L	20 L	20 L	25 L
61–80 kg	20 L	20 L	30 L	40 L
81–100 kg	20 L	25 L	40 L	50 L
101–120 kg	25 L	30 L	50 L	60 L
121–140 kg	25 L	40 L	50 L	

EOD, every other day.

maintain the cost of the therapy, decrease added burden of supply storage, and reduce the potential of increased utility costs to the patient. Typical clearances can be achieved with slow dialysate flow rates and with much less total dialysate per treatment than is normally used in the in-center setting. HD using the low dialysate flow rates achieves high fluid efficiency by optimizing the effective dwell time of the dialysate in the dialyzer. This occurs when the blood flow rate is high relative to the dialysate flow rate. Dialysate saturation exceeds 90% when the blood flow rate is approximately three times the dialysate flow rate. Total therapy volume per treatment is prescribed based on the patient's sex and weight. On average, patients that are 100 kg or less dialyzing five or six treatments per week can achieve clearance targets with 30 L per treatment or less. Lower treatment volumes decrease the amount of supply storage needed in the home and reduce home water utilization. Tables 4-1 and 4-2 demonstrate volume needs for more frequent dialysis with low-volume dialysate dialysis.

Dialysate volume needed to obtain a standard Kt/V (std Kt/V; also known as weekly std Kt/V) of 2.1 can be estimated and then adjusted based on biochemical findings. The single-pool Kt/V (sp Kt/V; also known as non equilibrated Kt/V) can be estimated based on days per week of therapy. For a standard Kt/V of 2.1, the sp Kt/V per treatment with 6 days is 0.44, 5 days is 0.6, 4 days is 0.8, and 3 days is 1.2.[17,18] Since the dialysate with low-flow dialysate is well saturated, the Kt would approximate the D/P urea × dialysate volume, and hence:

$$\frac{Kt}{V} = \frac{\frac{D}{P}\, \text{ratio} \times \text{dialysate volume}}{V}$$

$$\text{Dialysate volume} = \frac{\frac{Kt}{V} \times V}{\frac{D}{P}\, \text{ratio}}$$

where V = urea distribution volume, D/P ratio = dialysate-to-plasma ratio of urea.

Urea can be estimated to be 0.42 times body weight in females and 0.5 times body weight in males.[8] If the dialysate flow rate is near 1/3 of the blood flow rate, then the D/P ratio is 0.9. Hence for a male on 5 days per week of dialysis:

$$\text{Dialysate volume} = \frac{0.6 \times 0.5\,(\text{wt})}{0.9}$$

∎ BLOOD FLOW RATE AND VASCULAR ACCESS

Blood flow rate is an important determinate in achieving adequate dialysis. Most physicians prescribe the same blood flows as for conventional hemodialysis (CHD) in HHD. However, as with CHD, creating recirculation in a vascular access can lead to loss in therapy efficiency and alarms that interrupt treatment. Monitoring access pressures during treatment and ensuring that arterial pressure does not exceed −250 mm Hg helps to ensure appropriate use of the vascular access. Generally, higher blood flow rates such as 350 to 500 mL/min are appropriate for shorter treatments and lower blood flow rates such as 200 to 300 mL/min are appropriate for longer treatments such as nocturnal treatment.

[For more information, see Chapter 3.]

▌LACTATE VERSUS BICARBONATE-BASED DIALYSIS

Most conventional dialysis systems continue to utilize bicarbonate dialysate, which uses acetate as the acid concentrate. Prepackaged dialysate typically uses a lactate-based buffer. Precipitate does not form in lactate-based dialysate, unlike with bicarbonate solutions. Lactate also minimizes the chance of bacterial growth, as it can be stored safely for extended periods of time. Lactate is converted rapidly to bicarbonate on a 1:1 basis primarily by the liver and skeletal muscle. However, in patients with reduced lactate metabolism, it is important to carefully monitor tolerance of lactate-buffered dialysate. Lactate-based kinetics are not well studied but a recent study by Leypoldt et al. demonstrated less intradialytic and postdialytic alkalosis. Lactate levels are expected to rise during dialysis but decrease rapidly postdialysis as the lactate is converted. Lactate dose should be adjusted downward if there is predialysis alkalosis or upward if there is predialysis acidosis.[19]

▌POTASSIUM

Predialysis serum potassium concentrations should be monitored closely in HHD patients. A change in serum potassium may be experienced when transferring from CHD to more frequent HD. It is important to remember that changes in serum concentration are primarily a function of the dialysate potassium concentration and total dialysate volume per week. It should be noted however that low dialysate potassium concentrations when using large dialysate volume prescriptions may lead to large intradialytic reductions in serum potassium concentrations which can lead to excessively low postdialysis serum potassium concentrations. Utilizing lower dialysate volumes and lower dialysate flow rates will achieve a lower reduction in potassium concentrations than CHD. Therefore, low-volume dialysate prescriptions are prescribed with a 1 or a 2 mEq/L potassium concentration. This allows patients a slightly more liberal potassium diet. It should be noted that careful consideration should be taken with patients who dialyze nocturnally as potassium removal may be higher than those patients being treated with shorter treatment times.

▌EVALUATING DOSE OF HOME HEMODIALYSIS

Residual Renal Function

Literature suggests that there is a strong correlation between RRF and patient survival.[20] Preservation of RRF improves survival both in PD and potentially in HD patients. RRF is important for clearance of middle molecules, volume, and sodium removal. Attention should be placed on preserving RRF as well as ongoing monitoring of urine output. Efforts to preserve RRF in CKD patients include:

- Avoidance of nephrotoxic agents, especially aminoglycosides, non steroidal anti-inflammatory drugs, and cyclooxygenase-2 inhibitors
- Avoidance of excessive UF and hypotension during dialysis treatment
- Routine use of biocompatible dialyzer membranes
- Aggressive treatment of HTN
- Use of ACE inhibitors and ARBs as well as ultrapure dialysate

Monitoring RRF should at a minimum be done quarterly. The RRF urea clearance should be monitored closely if an adequate total Kt/V is reliant on urine Kt/V. At a minimum, RRF urea clearance should be monitored every 2 months, so prescriptions can be modified in the event of declining RRF. In general, it is acceptable to add the urea clearance from RRF and dialysis. An important caveat for the Centers for Medicare & Medicaid Services (CMS) is that in thrice-weekly dialysis, sp Kt/V should be >1.2 to 1.4 without the addition of RRF. Dialysate Kt/V is generally measured monthly in HD. In home patients, this is usually done in the home setting and the patient is trained on proper technique of pre- and post-blood urea nitrogen (BUN) collection. Additional data collected includes pre- and post weights to calculate UF, time of dialysis session, and frequency of dialysis performed.

Adjusting Prescriptions

The HHD prescription is often driven by target Kt/V, total body water, frequency, treatment time, and RRF. Kt/V, or urea clearance normalized to the patient's total body water, is the commonly used standard to determine adequacy of hemodialysis. sp Kt/V measures a per-treatment dose of HD by using pre-BUN and post-BUN levels and a conversion formula as described in K-DOQI. std Kt/V is a weekly dose of HD which was originally proposed by Gotch and has become a widely accepted measure of treatment frequencies four or greater times per week. Prescription adjustments need to be made when the Kt/V does not meet the target or clinical signs and symptoms indicated. The overall goals for successful HHD treatments are to achieve a std K/V greater than 2.1, phosphorus and middle molecule clearance, fluid removal with low UF rate, and QOL. Adjustments to the prescribed treatment are indicated when the patient's lifestyle requires changes to successfully complete treatments at home.

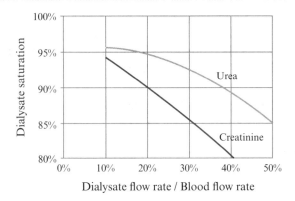

Figure 4-1 • Example of dialysate saturation with change in dialysate flow rate/blood flow rate.

One must first determine if the patient would benefit from an increase in treatment frequency or treatment length.

If treatment frequency is increased, the physician may have the opportunity to decrease the total volume of dialysate delivered during the treatment, therefore decreasing the total therapy time per treatment. However, patients may not be able to increase the frequency of treatments due to lifestyle limitations so increasing the therapy time per-treatment session could be a more suitable alternative.

Time can be increased by decreasing dialysate flow, which improves saturation (Kt) and increases time—this may be useful when Kt/V is within 10% of goal. Time also may be increased by increasing dialysate volume and maintaining consistent dialysate flow; this will improve clearance parallel to the increased volume of dialysate and increased time to use the dialysate prescribed. For example, in a situation with a dialysate flow rate of 200 mL/min, blood flow rate of 400 mL/min, and dialysate volume of 25 L, if dialysate flow decreases to 125 mL/min then saturation will rise from 87% to 94% (see Figure 4-1) and time will increase from 125 to 200 minutes. Kt/V will increase with improved clearance and increased time. If instead of decreasing dialysate flow, the dialysate volume increases to 30 L, maintaining dialysate flow 200 mL/min will increase clearance by 20% (increased dialysate volume 20%) and time will also increase from 125 to 150 minutes increasing Kt/V further. Once a prescription adjustment has been made, it is important to reevaluate the dose of dialysis within a week or two to ensure the prescription has achieved target.

[For more information, see Chapter 6.]

SOLO HOME HEMODIALYSIS

Solo HHD is defined as patients who chose to complete dialysis treatments in the home independently without a trained care partner for support. The benefit of solo HHD is that it allows more patients who might otherwise not be selected to do HHD to no longer be excluded from the modality due to lack of a care partner. The choice to do solo HHD should be a shared decision between the patient and the prescribing physician. Physicians should review the benefits and risks of solo HHD prior to training. Patients choosing to perform solo HHD must receive additional training to identify, avoid, or manage potential risks and complications of dialyzing alone. Patients performing solo HHD should be trained to utilize additional safety equipment during treatment such as a vascular access leak detector. Additional considerations when training solo HHD patients include evaluating the patient's ability to respond to alarms and troubleshoot complications independently, ability to perform all tasks required for a safe treatment at home with one hand, and notify emergency services when needed. Ideally, local emergency service personnel should be aware of the patient performing therapy and trained on emergency disconnection in the unlikely event of a medical emergency on dialysis.

[For more information, see Chapter 2.]

SUMMARY

HHD is dependent on HD device and design as well as prescription of dialysis. HD devices may change in the near future as new options become available. These devices must be reliable, minimize burden, allow telehealth monitoring, and provide economically viable and safe therapy with reliable delivery of care. Ideally, they should be flexible to allow appropriate individualization of therapy and portable if desired by the patient. Each device will also need to deliver safe and economic dialysate. The HHD prescription greatly impacts the patient's success on therapy. It is important to continuously evaluate the burden of HHD therapy. Prescriptions should be based on the patient's clinical needs and lifestyle. When the HHD prescription is individualized to meet the patient's needs, it provides quality dialysis and ensures technique retention.

REFERENCES

1. Liyanage T, Ninomiya T, Jha V. Worldwide access to treatment for end-stage kidney disease: a systematic review *Lancet*. 2015;385:1975-1982.

2. Weinhandl ED, Ray D, Kubisiak KM, Collins AJ. Contemporary trends in clinical outcomes among dialysis patients with Medicare coverage. *Am J Nephrol.* 2019;50:63-71.

3. Vinson AJ, Perl J, Tennankore KK. Survival comparisons of home dialysis versus in-center hemodialysis: a narrative review. *Can J Kidney Health Dis.* 2019;6:2054358119861941.

4. McCullough PA, Chan CT, Weinhandl ED, Burkart JM, Bakris GL. Intensive hemodialysis, left ventricular hypertrophy, and cardiovascular disease. *Am J Kidney Dis.* 2016;68(5S1):S5-S14.

5. Finkelstein FO, Schiller B, Daoui R, et al. At-home short daily hemodialysis improves the long-term health-related quality of life. *Kidney Int.* 2012;82:561-569.

6. Lacson E Jr, Xu J, Suri RS, et al. Survival with three-times weekly in-center nocturnal versus conventional hemodialysis. *J Am Soc Nephrol.* 2012;23(4):687-695.

7. Jaber BL, Lee Y, Collins AJ, et al. Effect of daily hemodialysis on depressive symptoms and postdialysis recovery time: interim report from the FREEDOM (Following Rehabilitation, Economics and Everyday-Dialysis Outcome Measurements) Study. *Am J Kidney Dis.* 2010;56:531-539.

8. Rocco MV, Lockridge RS Jr, Beck GJ, et al. The effects of frequent nocturnal home hemodialysis: The Frequent Hemodialysis Network Nocturnal Trial. *Kidney Int.* 2011;80(10):1080-1091.

9. Garofalo C, Borrelli S, De Stefano T, et al. Incremental dialysis in ESRD: systematic review and meta-analysis. *J Nephrol.* 2019;32(5):823-836.

10. Rhee CM, Unruh M, Chen J, Kovesdy CP, Zager P, Kalantar-Zadeh K. Infrequent dialysis: a new paradigm for hemodialysis initiation. *Semin Dial.* 2013;26(6):720-727.

11. Tennankore KK, Na Y, Wald R, et al. Short daily-, nocturnal- and conventional-home hemodialysis have similar patient and treatment survival. *Kidney Int.* 2018;93:188-194.

12. Woo KT, Choong HL, Foo MW, Tan HK, Wong KS, Chan CM. Survival with daily hemodialysis. *Kidney Int.* 2014;85(2):478-479.

13. Pierratos A. Nocturnal home hemodialysis: an update on a 5-year experience. *Nephrol Dial Transplant.* 1999;14:2835-2840.

14. Rayner HC, Zepel L, Fuller DS, et al. Recovery time, quality of life, and mortality in hemodialysis patients: the Dialysis Outcomes and Practice Patterns Study (DOPPS). *Am J Kidney Dis.* 2014;64(1):86-94.

15. Assimon MM, Wenger JB, Wang L, Flythe JE. Ultrafiltration rate and mortality in maintenance hemodialysis patients. *Am J Kidney Dis.* 2016;68(6):911-922.

16. Assimon MM, Flythe JE. Rapid ultrafiltration rates and outcomes among hemodialysis patients: re-examining the evidence base. *Curr Opin Nephrol Hypertens.* 2015;24(6):525-530.

17. Leypoldt JK, Jaber BL, Zimmerman DL. Predicting treatment dose for novel therapies using urea standard Kt/V. *Semin Dial.* 2004;17(2):142-145.

18. Daugirdas JT, Depner TA, Levin NW, Chertow GM, Rocco MV, FHN Trial Group. Standard Kt/V urea: a method of calculation that includes effects of fluid removal and residual renal clearance. *Kidney Int.* 2010;77(7):637-644.

19. Leypoldt JK, Pietribiasi M, Ebinger A, Kraus MA, Collins A, Waniewski J. Acid-base kinetics during hemodialysis using bicarbonate and lactate as dialysate buffer bases based on the H+ mobilization model. *Int J Artif Organs.* 2020;391398820906524. [Epub ahead of print, March 4, 2020]
20. Termorshuizen F. Relative contribution of residual renal function and different measures of adequacy to survival in hemodialysis patients: an analysis of the Netherlands Cooperative Study on the adequacy of dialysis. *J Am Soc Nephrol.* 2004;15(4):1061-1070.

5 WATER HANDLING IN HOME HEMODIALYSIS

Keiko I. Greenberg

OUTLINE

GENERAL CONSIDERATIONS
HOME HEMODIALYSIS MACHINES AND WATER PURIFICATION SYSTEMS
PLUMBING
WATER PURIFICATION
WATER QUALITY STANDARDS
MONITORING
COMPLICATIONS
SUMMARY

Water purification is crucial for hemodialysis (HD) as patients are exposed to large amounts of water with each treatment. Conventional hemodialysis (CHD) patients are typically exposed to more than 400 L of water each week, while for home hemodialysis (HHD) water exposure can vary from 150 L to significantly more than 400 L per week depending on the HD prescription and the dialysis system.[1] There are many substances that must be removed from the water supply to make it safe for dialysis. Water purification systems consist of a series of components that remove contaminants via different mechanisms. Regular monitoring of its components and of the product water is essential for ensuring proper function of the water system.[2] Failure to adequately treat the water supply can lead to serious adverse effects, including death.[3,4] While water standards are the same for CHD and HHD, some of the dialysis systems used for HHD differ from conventional machines. Water treatment is reviewed in this chapter with a focus on issues specific to HHD.

GENERAL CONSIDERATIONS

HHD can be done in nearly any home with electricity and water supply. A home visit should be conducted for any prospective patient to evaluate the suitability of the home for HHD. Testing of the water source to ensure it meets drinking water regulations or source water requirements is also necessary. In order to install a dialysis system in a home, some modifications must be made—these vary by the type of machine. Some homes may require alterations to the electrical supply, such as installation of a ground fault circuit interrupter outlet where the dialysis machine will be located in the home, or provision of a backup power supply.[5] Nearly all homes will require plumbing modifications. The costs associated with any modifications are borne by the dialysis provider and the patient does not incur any cost. If a patient does not own his or her home, such modifications must be approved by the landlord. Occasionally, a patient is unable to obtain permission to make modifications and therefore is unable to do HHD.

HOME HEMODIALYSIS MACHINES AND WATER PURIFICATION SYSTEMS

CHD machines are too large and heavy to be used in the home, and water purification systems for in-center HD units occupy very large spaces. HHD systems are scaled down in size and simplified for home use. The first machines used for HHD were conventional machines adapted for home use—an example of such a machine is Fresenius Medical Care's 2008K@ home HD machine, which is similar to its in-center HD machines in size and appearance.[6] It utilizes a separate reverse osmosis (RO) system for online water purification. More recently, machines designed specifically for HHD have been developed.[7] These include NxStage Medical Inc.'s System One, Quanta Dialysis Technologies Ltd.'s SC+, the Physidia S3 monitor, and Outset Medical Inc.'s Tablo system.[8,9] The vast majority of HHD patients in the United States use NxStage System One (Figure 5-1). Its water purification system is the PureFlow SL device, which uses deionization to make ultrapure water and then make dialysate in batches up to 60 L ahead of the dialysis treatment. Premixed bagged dialysate is also available for travel and for use as a backup to the PureFlow SL device. The Quanta SC+ uses RO for water purification and also has bagged dialysate available for travel. The Physidia S3 uses bagged dialysate only, so no water supply is needed. The Quanta SC+ and Physidia S3 are only

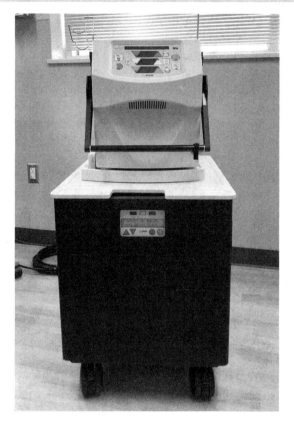

Figure 5-1 • The NxStage System One hemodialysis machine with PureFlow SL device. *(Photo courtesy of Arlene Hilario, RN.)*

available in Europe and are not available in the United States. In April 2020, Outset Medical, Inc. received clearance from the US Food and Drug Administration (FDA) for use of its Tablo system for HHD.[10] It has an integrated water purification system that uses RO.

▍PLUMBING

The water source for HD is typically a municipal water supply, but may be a well or other source, particularly in rural areas. The water supply may be from a bathroom or laundry room. All dialysis systems (except for the Physidia S3, which uses bagged dialysate only) require a supply line and a waste line (Figure 5-2) and these alone may be sufficient to install the PureFlow SL device for the NxStage system. For systems that use RO for water purification, additional modifications may be necessary. A booster pump or other equipment may be necessary to ensure adequate water

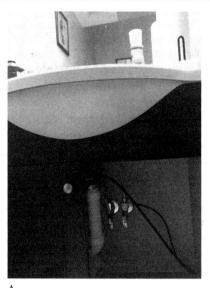
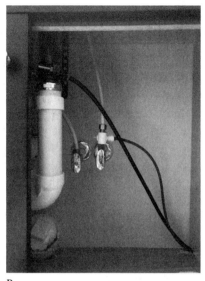

A   B

Figure 5-2 • Example of plumbing for HHD with a supply line and waste line. Water and waste line installation for NxStage PureFlow SL system under bathroom vanity (A). Closer view (B). *(Photos courtesy of Arlene Hilario, RN.)*

pressure for RO machines.[5] Backflow preventers that keep water from being forced from the RO machine back to the water supply are required in some countries. Devices that control water temperature may also be needed if source water is not at an appropriate temperature. Regardless of the specific plumbing modifications that are required, these should be carried out by an experienced plumber familiar with dialysis systems.

▌WATER PURIFICATION

Many substances and contaminants are found in municipal water at levels suitable for drinking but not for HD use. These include[11]:

- Substances added to improve water quality including chlorine/chloramines, fluoride, and aluminum
- Metals that may leach from plumbing systems including lead and copper
- Trace elements naturally occurring in the water
- Organic matter
- Agricultural products including nitrates and fertilizers
- Microorganisms including bacteria, fungi, and protozoa and endotoxins

Known toxicities associated with specific contaminants are listed in Table 5-1.[11] In addition, exposure to microorganisms can lead to serious systemic infections. Endotoxin exposure causes acute symptoms such as fever, chills, nausea, myalgias, weakness, headache, hypotension and shock (known as pyrogenic reactions), and long-term complications, primarily β2-microglobulin amyloidosis.[12]

Each water purification system requires multiple components to generate water for HD. These components include filters, water softeners, carbon tanks/beds, RO systems, deionizers, and ultraviolet light.[1] Filters include multimedia or sediment filters that remove particulate debris found in source water at the start of the purification process, cartridge filters that remove fine particles from carbon tanks, and endotoxin retentive filters that remove bacteria and endotoxins. If a nonmunicipal water supply is used for HHD, the specific filters needed are determined by analyzing the water supply.[13] Poor quality of the water supply can negatively impact the function and durability of RO membranes and carbon filters. Water softeners remove calcium and magnesium in areas with "hard" water to protect RO membranes—this occurs via ion exchange

Table 5-1	SIGNS AND SYMPTOMS OF WATER CONTAMINATION
Contaminant	**Signs and Symptoms of Exposure**
Aluminum	Intoxication, seizures, neurologic symptoms, bone disease, anemia
Calcium	Confusion, lethargy, nausea, vomiting
Copper	Hemolysis, acidosis, nausea, seizure, shock
Chlorine/Chloramines	Hemolysis, methemoglobinemia
Fluoride	Intoxication, pruritus, headache, nausea, chest pain, ventricular fibrillation
Lead	Neuropathy, anemia, abdominal pain, confusion, seizures
Nitrate	Methemoglobinemia, cyanosis
Sodium	Hypertension, thirst, pulmonary edema, confusion, seizure
Sulfate	Nausea, vomiting, chills, fever
Zinc	Nausea, vomiting, fever, anemia

where cations are replaced with sodium ions.[1] Carbon tanks and beds contain activated carbon granules that remove chorine and chloramine via adsorption. RO systems remove metal ions, organic and inorganic solutes, bacteria, endotoxins, and viruses by utilizing high pressures to force water through a semipermeable membrane. Deionization systems remove cations and anions using exchange resins. Ultraviolet lights kill free microbes in the water.

An example configuration of a water purification system for a CHD machine adapted to home use is shown in Figure 5-3.[14] RO systems may require a booster pump to ensure adequate water pressure and/or temperature blending valve to ensure adequate water temperature, as RO function decreases with lower temperatures.[13] Water and electricity usage are significant for RO systems. They also require regular disinfection. The NxStage PureFlow SL system does not utilize RO—it includes a sediment filter, ultraviolet light, carbon media, dual deionization beds, resistivity sensors that monitor water quality after each deionization bed, endotoxin retentive ultrafilters, and a 0.2 micron filter (Figure 5-4).[14] The disposable purification pack (PAK) is replaced every 12 weeks or earlier if the deionization resins are exhausted. No disinfection is needed.

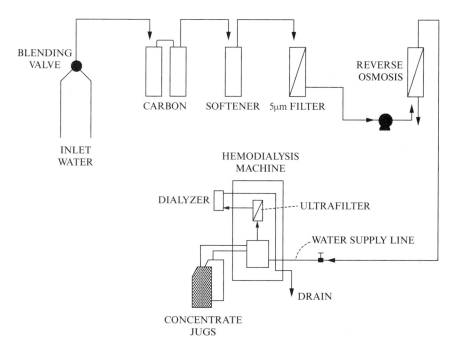

Figure 5-3 • Example of a water treatment system for conventional machine adapted for HHD. *(Reproduced with permission from Ouseph R, Ward RA. Ultrapure Dialysate for Home Hemodialysis? Adv Chronic Kidney Dis. 2007;14(3):256-62. Copyright © National Kidney Foundation, Inc. Published by Elsevier, Inc. All rights reserved. https://www.ackdjournal.org/.)*

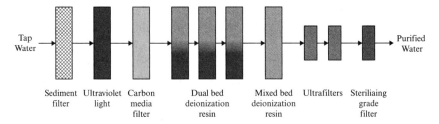

Figure 5-4 • The components of the PureFlow Purification Pack (PAK). *(From NxStage Medical, Inc. Therapy Handbook NxStage® Hemodialysis Treatment. https://www.nxstage. com/wp-content/uploads/2019/08/NxStage-Hemodialysis-Treatment-Therapy-Handbook. pdf. Updated August 2019. Accessed January 8, 2020.)*

WATER QUALITY STANDARDS

The water produced by purification systems must meet guidelines published by the American National Standards Institute (ANSI) and the Association for the Advancement of Medical Instrumentation (AAMI) or the International Organization for Standardization (ISO). Maximum allowable concentrations of 22 contaminants are listed in Table 5-2.[15] Maximal allowable bacteria counts and endotoxin levels are shown in Table 5-3. If either bacteria counts or endotoxin level reach an "action level" of 50% of the maximum allowable level, then action must be taken to implement procedures to prevent further increase.[15] Most HHD systems are able to produce ultrapure water, which has a bacterial total viable count <0.1 CFU/mL and endotoxin levels <0.03 EU/mL. The use of ultrapure water has increased in recent years due to concerns that microbial contaminants in dialysate cause chronic inflammation.[13,14] It has been associated with reduction in use of erythropoiesis-stimulating agents (ESAs), reduction in macroglobulin, increase in serum albumin, and preservation of residual renal function (RRF), although it is unknown whether it improves mortality.[13,14]

[For more information, see Chapter 7.]

MONITORING

Protocols for monitoring of source water, dialysate water, and dialysate vary by type of water purification system and clinic. Chlorine testing is typically done with every treatment or batch of dialysate, but other chemical monitoring may occur less frequently in HHD than in the in-center setting.[16,17] Bacterial contamination is, fortunately, a lesser concern in HHD due to the short length of pipes compared to lengthy distribution loops in dialysis units; therefore, bacterial cultures and endotoxin testing are often

Table 5-2 MAXIMUM ALLOWABLE CONCENTRATION OF CONTAMINANTS IN DIALYSIS WATER		
Contaminant		**AAMI Standard (mg/L)**
Contaminants with documented toxicity in HD patients	Aluminum	0.01
	Total chlorine	0.1
	Copper	0.1
	Fluoride	0.2
	Lead	0.005
	Nitrate (as N)	2
	Sulfate	100
	Zinc	0.1
Electrolytes normally included in dialysis fluid	Calcium	2 (0.05 mmol/L)
	Magnesium	4 (0.15 mmol/L)
	Potassium	8 (0.2 mmol/L)
	Sodium	70 (3.0 mmol/L)
Trace elements	Antimony	0.006
	Arsenic	0.005
	Barium	0.1
	Beryllium	0.0004
	Cadmium	0.001
	Chromium	0.014
	Mercury	0.0002
	Selenium	0.09
	Silver	0.005
	Thallium	0.002

© ISO. This material is adapted from *ANSI/AAMI/ISO 23500-3:2019*, with permission of the American National Standards Institute (ANSI) on behalf of the International Organization for Standardization. All rights reserved.

done less frequently than in the dialysis center.[13] Effective patient training and adherence to monitoring and equipment maintenance are crucial for the performance of safe HD.

[For more information, see Chapter 6.]

Table 5-3 MAXIMAL ALLOWABLE LEVELS FOR BACTERIA AND ENDOTOXIN			
	Dialysis Water	Standard Dialysis Fluid	Ultrapure Dialysis Fluid
TVC (CFU/mL)	<100	<100	<0.1
Endotoxin (EU/mL)	<0.25	<0.5	<0.03

CFU, colony-forming units; EU, endotoxin units; TVC, total viable count.

© ISO. This material is adapted from *ANSI/AAMI/ISO 23500-5:2019*, with permission of the American National Standards Institute (ANSI) on behalf of the International Organization for Standardization. All rights reserved.

▌COMPLICATIONS

Improper maintenance of the water purification system or malfunction of any of its components could lead to contaminant exposure and serious clinical consequences. In the United States, there were 13 incidents of chemical intoxication affecting nearly 200 HD patients between 1960 and 2007.[3] These included[3]:

- Aluminum intoxication
- Hemolytic anemia due to chloramine
- Hemolytic anemia due to copper
- Fluoride intoxication
- Formaldehyde intoxication
- Anemia due to hydrogen peroxide
- Severe hypotension due to sodium azide
- Nausea, vomiting, chills, fevers due to sulfates

One of these incidents involved a patient on HHD who used a well for his water supply.[3,18] A few months after starting HHD, he developed nausea, vomiting, lethargy, weakness, and hypotension. He was cyanotic on presentation and his blood was noted to be brown. He was presumed to have methemoglobinemia and treated with methylene blue with improvement in his condition. His well water was found to have an extremely high nitrate concentration of 94 mg/L. He was able to resume HHD after installation of a water deionizer. It is important to note that levels of some contaminants, including nitrates, in the water supply can vary with weather conditions.[4]

HHD patients may be at higher risk of chloramine exposure and resultant anemia due to use of smaller carbon filters with RO systems. A study in the United Kingdom showed that switching HHD patients to a larger size carbon filter reduced ESA requirements.[4] In addition to the incidents involving chemical intoxication, there were 20 events caused by bacterial or endotoxin (or both) contamination between 1960 and 2007.[3] About half of the events occurred in the setting of dialyzer reuse. As mentioned previously, the risk of bacterial contamination in HHD is lower than with CHD, and pyrogenic reactions in HHD are rare.[13] Excessively high dialysate temperature can result in hemolysis—this is very unlikely to occur with current dialysis machines that alarm when temperatures are too high.[19]

In the event that dialysis water does not meet guidelines, or there is a malfunction of the water purification system, the water should not be used for dialysis. Premixed bagged dialysate should be used for systems that have this option.

[For more information, see Chapter 8.]

▌SUMMARY

Water treatment is a critical component of HD. Water treatment systems for HHD may use RO systems like in HD clinics, or use deionization, or avoid the need to make dialysate altogether by using premixed bagged dialysate. Some electrical and plumbing modifications may be required to install HHD systems in the home. Adequate patient training, monitoring of water quality, and maintenance of HHD systems are crucial for performing safe and effective HD.

▌REFERENCES

1. Ahmad S. Essentials of water treatment in hemodialysis. *Hemodial Int.* 2005;9(2):127-134.
2. Kasparek T, Rodriguez OE. What medical directors need to know about dialysis facility water management. *Clin J Am Soc Nephrol.* 2015;10(6):1061-1071.
3. Coulliette AD, Arduino MJ. Hemodialysis and water quality. *Semin Dial.* 2013;26(4):427-438.
4. Davenport A. Complications of hemodialysis treatments due to dialysate contamination and composition errors. *Hemodial Int.* 2015;19(suppl 3):S30-3.
5. Agar JW, Perkins A, Heaf JG. Home hemodialysis: infrastructure, water, and machines in the home. *Hemodial Int.* 2015;19(suppl 1):S93-S111.
6. Schlaeper C, Diaz-Buxo JA. The Fresenius Medical Care home hemodialysis system. *Semin Dial.* 2004;17(2):159-161.
7. Haroon S, Davenport A. Haemodialysis at home: review of current dialysis machines. *Expert Rev Med Devices.* 2018;15(5):337-347.

8. Clark WR, Turk JE Jr. The NxStage System One. *Semin Dial*. 2004;17(2):167-170.

9. Harasemiw O, Day C, Milad JE, Grainger J, Ferguson T, Komenda P. Human factors testing of the Quanta SC+ hemodialysis system: an innovative system for home and clinic use. *Hemodial Int*. 2019;23(3):306-313.

10. Outset Medical Inc. Tablo® Hemodialysis System receives FDA clearance for home dialysis. Outset Medical. Available at https://www.outsetmedical.com/news/tablo-hemodialysis-system-receives-fda-clearance-for-home-dialysis/. Accessed April 21, 2020.

11. Bieber S. Water treatment equipment for in-center hemodialysis. In: Nissenson AR, Fine RN, eds. *Handbook of Dialysis Therapy*. 5th ed. Philadelphia, PA: Elsevier; 2017:chap 10.

12. Brunet P, Berland Y. Water quality and complications of haemodialysis. *Nephrol Dial Transplant*. 2000;15(5):578-580.

13. Damasiewicz MH, Polkinghorne KR, Kerr PG. Water quality in conventional and home haemodialysis. *Nat Rev Nephrol*. 2012;8(12):725-734.

14. Ouseph R, Ward RA. Ultrapure dialysate for home hemodialysis? *Adv Chronic Kidney Dis*. 2007;14(3):256-262.

15. American National Standards Institute, Inc., Association for the Advancement of Medical Instrumentation, and International Organization for Standardization. ANSI/AAMI/ISO 23500-3:2019, Preparation and quality management of fluids for haemodialysis and related therapies—part 3: water for haemodialysis and related therapies. Available at https://www.aami.org. Accessed June 26, 2020.

16. NxStage Medical, Inc. *Therapy Handbook: NxStage Hemodialysis Treatment*. Available at https://www.nxstage.com/wp-content/uploads/2019/08/NxStage-Hemodialysis-Treatment-Therapy-Handbook.pdf. Updated August 2019. Accessed January 8, 2020.

17. Fresenius Medical Care. 2008K@home User's Guide, 490180 Revision G. Available at https://fmcna.com/content/dam/fmcna/live/support/documents/operator's-manuals---hemodialysis-(hd)/2008k%40home-operator's-manuals/490180_Rev_G.pdf. Updated March 1, 2018. Accessed January 10, 2020.

18. Carlson DJ, Shapiro FL. Methemoglobinemia from well water nitrates: a complication of home dialysis. *Ann Intern Med*. 1970;73(5):757-759.

19. Saha M, Allon M. Diagnosis, treatment, and prevention of hemodialysis emergencies. *Clin J Am Soc Nephrol*. 2017;12(2):357-369.

LABORATORY PARAMETERS AND MONITORING FOR HOME HEMODIALYSIS

6

Cynthia Christiano and J. Clint Parker

The goal of every home hemodialysis (HHD) program should be to provide safe, quality care; this cannot be accomplished without routine monitoring. Monitoring involves the systematic observation of particular parameters in order to *discover* disease, adverse outcomes, or risk factors or to *assess* interventions aimed at treatment, prevention, or reduction of risk. In this chapter, we will begin by discussing three basic questions involved in monitoring. We will then focus on population monitoring in an HHD unit as exemplified through the quality assurance and improvement (QAI) process, and lastly, we will discuss examples of individual patient monitoring utilizing recommendations from national guidelines.

▌ THREE BASIC QUESTIONS

When thinking about monitoring, three basic questions arise:

1. What is being monitored?
2. Who is being monitored?
3. Why is monitoring being done?

What Is Being Monitored?

Monitoring can be used to screen for disease, adverse outcomes, or risk factors. For example, dialysis units periodically screen patients for hepatitis, anemia, hyperphosphatemia, and malnutrition irrespective of whether patients currently have these conditions. However, many patients do develop these conditions and require the initiation of therapy. In these cases, monitoring is used to access the efficacy of ongoing treatment. Typically, goals of therapy involve maintaining particular parameters inside prespecified ranges.

Monitoring, however, goes beyond laboratory testing. Non-laboratory monitoring is common for disease screening, assessment of therapy, prevention efforts, and risk reduction efforts. Common examples of non-laboratory screening include blood pressure monitoring for non-hypertensive patients, depression screening, and access monitoring via physical exam and access flow measurement. Examples of monitoring of therapeutic interventions include periodic depression surveys to assess depression treatment and blood pressure measuring for hypertensive patients. It is also vital to monitor the success of the dialysis therapy itself. To do so, we use both laboratory parameters (i.e., urea reduction ratio [URR] and Kt/V) and non-laboratory parameters (i.e., intradialytic weight gains, flowsheet monitoring, etc.).

Who Is Being Monitored?

Generally, there are two perspectives one might take with regards to monitoring: a patient perspective and a population perspective.

Patient Perspective

The patient perspective involves monitoring individual patients in order to discover disease, adverse outcomes, or risk factors and in order to assess interventions aimed at treatment, prevention, or reduction of risk. This perspective is fundamental. The interdisciplinary team (IDT) consisting of physicians, nurses, dialysis technicians, dieticians, and social workers evaluate and balance the multiple and sometimes competing therapeutic goals that exist in a particular patient at a particular time with all the unique exigencies and values that individual patients bring to a clinic encounter. Careful balancing must be done to achieve the optimal outcome. For example, in a patient who is exhibiting signs of malnourishment, the IDT may liberalize dietary restrictions even if this leads to a mildly elevated phosphorous level. The patient perspective utilizes all the results of monitoring in order to arrive at an individualized clinical plan that is optimal for a particular patient.

Population Perspective

The population perspective, however, operates differently. During QAI sessions, physicians, clinic managers, and dialysis personnel evaluate the results of monitoring for the dialysis population as a whole. The focus is not on individual patients but on the group. The questions are significantly different. From a population perspective, one wants to know what percentage of the population has met predefined goals for the parameters being monitored. For example, the hemoglobin goal for individual patients on erythropoietin-stimulating agent (ESA) therapy may be 10 to 11.5 g/dL, but one would also want to know what percentage of one's dialysis population is actually meeting this goal and how that percentage compares to benchmarks.

Why Is Monitoring Being Done?

The goals of monitoring from an individual patient perspective involve both screening and assessment. The goals of monitoring from a population perspective are to identify trends with regards to the presence, management, prevention, and reduction of disease, adverse outcomes, and risk factors in order to identify systemic problems that would be amenable to formalized quality improvement initiatives. These initiatives help identify solutions to problems that can be implemented in a systematic manner to improve care. For example, through its routine population monitoring, a dialysis unit may note that its percentage of patients with dialysis catheters has increased. This knowledge would trigger a quality improvement initiative to investigate why the percentage of dialysis catheters has increased and to identify strategies to reduce the catheter rate. Providers can then use these strategies as they formulate individual care plans for patients. In what follows, we will detail population monitoring for HHD patients as it occurs within the QAI process.

POPULATION MONITORING THROUGH THE QUALITY ASSURANCE AND IMPROVEMENT PROCESS

Defining Quality

Before moving forward with specifics concerning HHD, it is important to define quality as it pertains to healthcare. According to the Institute of Medicine, healthcare quality is defined as "the degree to which health care services for individuals and populations increase the likelihood of desired health outcomes and are consistent with current professional knowledge."[1] To further expand on this definition, six different domains of quality have been outlined (Table 6-1).[1]

When first entering the world of quality, it is easy to be overwhelmed. However, remember that quality is not a destination, but a journey. We

Table 6-1 INSTITUTE OF MEDICINE QUALITY DOMAINS	
Effectiveness	Relates to providing care processes and achieving outcomes as supported by scientific evidence.
Efficiency	Relates to maximizing the quality of a comparable unit of healthcare delivered or unit of health benefit achieved for a given unit of healthcare resources used.
Equity	Relates to providing healthcare of equal quality to those who may differ in personal characteristics other than their clinical condition or preferences for care.
Patient centeredness	Relates to meeting patients' needs and preferences and providing education and support.
Safety	Relates to actual or potential bodily harm.
Timeliness	Relates to obtaining needed care while minimizing delays.

Reproduced with permission from Understanding Quality Measurement. Content last revised October 2018. Agency for Healthcare Research and Quality, Rockville, MD. https://www.ahrq.gov/patient-safety/quality-resources/tools/chtoolbx/understand/index.html.

should always be striving to achieve better outcomes in all aspects of patient care, and one way to accomplish this is through QAI. Simply put, QAI is a process that involves the following steps:

1. Identify an area needing improvement and establish a goal
2. Determine the root cause or causes as to why performance in that area is suboptimal
3. Brainstorm to develop solutions
4. Gather resources available to help execute the developed solutions
5. Implement the plan
6. Determine whether improvement occurred
7. Analyze the findings

These general QAI principles and steps can be translated into meaningful projects pertinent to the end-stage kidney disease (ESKD) population. There are several templates available to help with this process including the toolkits developed by the Medical Advisory Council of the National Forum of ESRD Networks.[2]

Quality Monitoring Team

Routine QAI consisting of both administrative and clinical oversight is a central component of every effective HHD program. Although quality monitoring is a daily, ongoing process, each program should have a quality monitoring team (QAI team) that meets on a regular basis. In fact, the success of an HHD program often depends on the commitment and engagement of the QAI team, and the team's infrastructure is thought to be one of the most important components of any home dialysis program.[3] This quality structure is not only necessary for the success of the program, but is mandated by the Centers for Medicare & Medicaid Services (CMS). This is the governmental agency responsible for surveying and certifying ESKD facilities for inclusion in the Medicare Program. To be included facilities must meet specified safety and quality standards, called Conditions for Coverage (CfC). The Survey and Certification Program provides initial certification of new dialysis facilities as well as ongoing monitoring to ensure that these facilities continue to meet these basic requirements.[4]

CfC regulation 494.110 V626 states, "the dialysis facility must develop, implement, maintain, and evaluate an effective, data-driven, quality assessment and performance improvement program with participation by the professional members of the interdisciplinary team."[5] At a minimum, this team should consist of the program's administrator, medical director, clinical manager, registered nurse, technician, social worker, and dietician. It is also of benefit to have additional nursing and support staff present. The meetings should be at least monthly, but more often as the need arises. The main focus of the meeting is not to review each patient individually but to ensure that the program is providing safe, quality care. To accomplish this goal, the QAI team should review important topics on a regular basis. The elements of an HHD quality assurance meeting are outlined in Table 6-2. In what follows we will briefly review each of these topics.

Program Overview

The overarching goals of an HHD program should be safety, quality, and growth. An in-depth program overview is necessary to set the framework for monitoring these parameters. It allows the QAI team to understand the program's current status as well as set specific goals for the future. Patient census, training outcomes, attrition rates, and interdisciplinary staffing ratios should be reviewed. A successful program should aim to train at least one patient per month with a goal of maintaining at least 20 active patients.[6] However, safety and quality should never be sacrificed for growth. A unit committed to providing excellent patient care will grow in time. Adequate staffing is an essential part of that equation and will impact every aspect of the program. The importance of committed, experienced staff cannot be over emphasized. Another area to remember

Table 6-2   ELEMENTS OF AN HHD QUALITY ASSURANCE MEETING

Program Overview
- Census for both patients and staff
- Growth plan for patients, staff, and space
- Training success rate
- Patient attrition rate and reason
- High-risk patient discussion (both existing and proposed patients)

Regulatory Overview
- Policy and procedures
- Survey review (when applicable)
- Care plan review including quality of life surveys
- Emergency preparedness

Technical Review
- Water quality
- Equipment recalls

Adverse Events/Patient Grievances
- Serious event review/Root cause determination/Action plan development
- Infection tracking

Population-Based Patient Monitoring
- Laboratory monitoring
- Non-laboratory monitoring

when monitoring a program is clinical space. Adequate space is needed for effective training, interdisciplinary meetings, and clinic visits. Space is particularly important to consider when developing growth goals.

[For more information, see Chapter 15.]

Patient Recruitment and Retention

The process of providing and monitoring quality care starts with patient recruitment. With the increasing interest in HHD, some believe that all patients should be offered the opportunity to utilize this modality. However, practical considerations do exist and it is the responsibility of the QAI team to have an ongoing review of current patients as well as to discuss the suitability of potential patients. Home visits are an important part of this process and should be done at a minimum prior to training, after each adverse event, and with any change in patient status. Checklists are helpful to ensure that the patient's home is evaluated for cleanliness, appropriate space, and technical concerns. This is also an opportunity to provide additional education to the patient, family, and care partner. Program standards for patient selection, home visits, and training should be developed and reviewed on a regular basis.

Since observational studies have demonstrated an association between intensive HHD and lower risk of death as well as increased patient-reported quality of life (QOL) and independence, every attempt should be made to help patients interested in HHD succeed.[7,8] If patients are committed and motivated, most barriers can be overcome. Some of the more common barriers preventing patients from being suited for and successful at HHD are poor personal hygiene, frailty, hearing impairments, and illiteracy. Hygiene education, dialysis partner training, patient physiotherapy, occupational therapy, multimedia training, as well as utilization of vibration/light alarms are suggested interventions.[3] The QAI team should oversee these efforts and monitor the program's training outcomes with special attention to high-risk patients. Training takes a significant amount of time and effort, with most programs training patients for 4 to 6 weeks. Therefore, it is in the program's best interest for this time to be productive and successful. Training is considered a success if the patient is able to safely and effectively perform his treatments at home. If a training endeavor is not successful, a root cause should be determined and the information brought to the QAI team meeting for review and discussion.

Effective, high-quality programs should not only focus on the number of patients successfully trained but also on the number of patients maintained on HHD. It is important to remember that growth only occurs when a program is able to retain its current patients at home. Therefore, patient attrition should be a focal point of the program overview. Understanding why patients are discharged from the program is necessary for quality improvement. The goal is to have discharges secondary only to transplantation. However, physical and social changes may occur that prevent patients from safely performing treatment at home. These barriers to HHD should be identified and overcome if possible.

Another reason why patients abandon home dialysis is patient and care partner burnout. A systemic review of this topic revealed that the QOL of care partners of dialysis recipients is poorer than the general population. However, the impact of caring for HHD patients has not been well studied.[9] The program should strive to recognize patients and care partners at risk for burnout and implement coping and support strategies.

[For more information, see Chapters 2, 7, and 8.]

Regulatory Overview

Although this chapter is focused primarily on the clinical monitoring of an HHD program, it is necessary to recognize that dialysis facilities must have and abide by its policies and procedures. It is the responsibility of the QAI team to approve the policies and procedures and continuously monitor them for relevance and medical accuracy. In addition, dialysis facilities must abide by state and national regulations. The QAI team must understand these regulations and ensure that the program is in compliance. For example, personnel licensing and ongoing training requirements must be reviewed and kept up-to-date. Reimbursement rules must be understood to allow appropriate payments for both the facility and the nephrologist. All of these requirements are of particular importance when starting a de novo center. Establishing a new HHD program can be an extremely rewarding endeavor, but does take knowledge, resources, and patience. The International Society of Hemodialysis has a Home Dialysis Toolkit for implementing hemodialysis (HD) in the home, which can serve as an excellent resource.[10]

[For more information, see Chapter 15.]

Survey Review

Centers for Medicare & Medicaid Services Surveys

CMS provides regulatory oversight for dialysis care in the United States through survey and certification programs. CMS survey results should be carefully reviewed at the QAI meeting and corrective action plans developed as needed. The QAI team should strive to have the program "survey ready" at all times or in other words be in compliance with all CfC regulations. To achieve this, regulatory and clinical audits should be conducted on a regular basis. This should include chart audits, personnel file audits, technical audits, inventory audits, and infection control audits. The results of these audits should be presented at the QAI meeting along with any action plans needed to improve compliance.

Patient Satisfaction Surveys

The patient satisfaction survey helps to gauge the dialysis unit's performance in providing the patient with the best possible dialysis experience. It allows the QAI team to see the program through the eyes of the patients and should be reviewed in detail at the QAI meeting. Areas of excellence for the program should be celebrated and areas needing improvement should be addressed. An overview of the results of the survey and ways the program plans to change in response to the survey should be shared with patients.

Independent of these surveys, each program should have a process in place for patient feedback and grievances. The program should strive to provide an environment in which patients feel comfortable and safe expressing concerns. Each concern should be brought to the attention of the QAI team so that resolution plans can be developed and outcomes can be monitored.

Care Planning

Care planning on each patient is an additional regulatory requirement worth mentioning. When done correctly, this process can be a meaningful part of patient care. Care planning is exactly what the name implies; it is a process that allows every discipline to review the patient's care in detail and develop strategies for quality improvement. Patients, family members, and care partners are invited to the meeting and encouraged to participate. Care plans should be done within 30 days of admission to the program, again at 90 days, and then annually as long as the patient is deemed stable by the IDT. If the patient is felt to be unstable, the care plan should be conducted monthly until the patient's condition improves. Along with the care plans, a QOL survey should be administered to the patient and referrals made for psychological support as indicated. It is the responsibility of the QAI team to ensure that care plans and QOL surveys are being administered per policy.

Emergency Preparedness

Oversight of emergency preparedness is another requirement of the QAI team. All patients should be registered with the local water and power companies so they are aware of the need to restore services as soon as possible if a disruption does occur. In addition, a risk assessment should be done annually. This is a process that identifies potential hazards and analyzes what could happen if the hazard indeed occurs. There are several risk assessment tools available. The QAI team should establish a relationship with local emergency management services and draw from their expertise in this area. Patients should be educated as to what to do in emergency situations. They should be advised to keep at least 2 weeks of medication and dialysis supplies on hand. They should check the expiration date on their dialysis supplies on a regular basis. In addition, they should have an evacuation plan that can be executed quickly if needed. Emergency packets should be distributed to each patient at least annually and as needed depending on potential natural disasters. These packets should include patient-specific information such as a list of medical conditions, medications, and allergies along with a prescription for a potassium-lowering agent in case the dialysis schedule is interrupted. In addition, emergency phone numbers and general emergency preparedness information should be included. CMS has an excellent resource entitled, Preparing for Emergencies: A Guide for People on Dialysis.[11]

Technical Review

A technician should be present at all QAI meetings to present an overview of technical-related HHD issues. This should include water testing, machine updates, and equipment recalls.

[For more information, see Chapter 5.]

Adverse Events

Serious Safety Events

Although successful HHD has been done for decades in the United States, concerns about the safety of home dialysis are often expressed by potential HHD patients and family members. These concerns are often centered on the dialysis procedure itself. It is important to understand and be able to convey that HHD is a safe dialysis modality and serious adverse events are rare. Yet, it is the responsibility of the QAI team to recognize potential causes of serious adverse events, ensure that policies and procedures are in place to safeguard against these events, and review in detail all events and near misses that do occur.

In a quality assurance perspective study of two HHD programs in Canada, one death and six potentially fatal adverse events were noted to occur during a 12-year period.[12] This translated into a crude death rate of 2 per 1000 patient-years and a cumulative life-threatening procedure-related adverse event rate of approximately 14 events per 1000 patient-years.[13] Of the seven events that were reported, blood loss due to human error was the immediate cause of the adverse event in six cases. This highlights the importance of initial training as well as ongoing training updates. All lessons learned from serious adverse events and near misses should be incorporated into the training curriculum. A list of potential procedure-related adverse events as well as a prevention plan is outlined in Table 6-3.[12]

Despite preventative measures, vigilant training, and adherence to policies and procedures, serious adverse events, although rare, will occur. The response of the patient and the program can affect the outcome of the current event as well as occurrences and outcomes of future events. Patients should be educated on emergency procedures and these should be practiced on a regular basis. The simple "clamp-and-call" plan is one such emergency procedure (Figure 6-1).[13]

Patients should also be advised to keep a folder with basic information near the dialysis machine at all times. This folder should be labeled

Table 6-3 POTENTIAL HHD ADVERSE EVENTS	
Adverse Event	**Prevention Plan**
Exsanguination into the circuit	Priming and rinse-back procedures to make it impossible to bleed into circuit by eliminating disconnection and reconnection of arterial and/or venous tubing to/from patient
Exsanguination from the circuit	Unimpeded placement of wetness detectors in correct positions; ensure proper threading and integrity of connectors
Exsanguination from the access	Placement of wetness detectors in correct positions; use of closed connector devices (for CVCs); ensure proper placement of clamps (for CVCs)
Air embolism	Use of closed connector devices (for CVCs)
Inadvertent hemodynamic decompensation due to ultrafiltration	Increase frequency and duration of treatments to decrease overall ultrafiltration rate; continued education regarding salt and water intake (particularly important because patients may have the false assumption that intensive HD absolves them of dietary restrictions); regular careful assessment of patient's dry weight; consider a care partner requirement; lower dialysate temperature; avoid intradialytic food ingestion
Inadvertent hemodynamic decompensation from dialysate leak	Placement of wetness detectors; ensure proper threading of dialysate tubing to dialyzer
Hemolysis	Ensure absence of kinks in tubing; regular monitoring of water quality

CVC, central venous catheter; HD, hemodialysis.

Reproduced with permission from Wong B, Zimmerman D, Reinties F, et al. Procedure-related serious adverse events among home hemodialysis patients: A quality assurance perspective. *Am J Kidney Dis.* 2013;63:251-258. Copyright © 2014 National Kidney Foundation, Inc. Published by Elsevier, Inc. All rights reserved. https://www.sciencedirect.com/journal/american-journal-of-kidney-diseases.

for emergency medical services (EMS) use and should include emergency contact information, dialysis facility contact information, a list of medical conditions, a list of current medications, and a letter to EMS and emergency room personnel.[13] An example of this is shown in Table 6-4.

Once a serious adverse event occurs, the clinical manager and medical director should be notified immediately. Certain processes should occur that will help determine the root cause of the event and hopefully

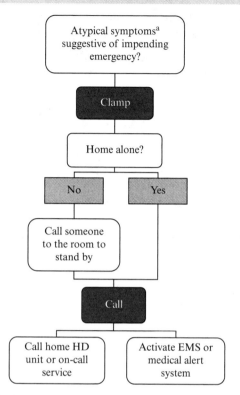

Figure 6-1 • Home hemodialysis "clamp-and-call" emergency management algorithm. [a] Atypical symptoms include but are not limited to presyncope, heart palpitations, chest pressure, focal neurological symptoms, or deteriorating level of consciousness. EMS, emergency medical services; HD, hemodialysis. (*Reproduced with permission from Pauly RP, Eastwood DO, Marshall MR. Patient safety in home hemodialysis: Quality assurance and serious adverse events in the home setting. Hemodial Int. 2015;19(Supp 1):S59-S70. Copyright © John Wiley and Sons.*)

prevent further events from taking place. These processes are outlined in Table 6-5.[12] All of these steps should be reviewed at the QAI meeting. If needed, policies and procedures should be updated and training curriculum changed.

[For more information, see Chapter 8.]

Dialysis-Associated Infections

Infection control oversight is another requirement of the QAI team and infection control principles should be discussed with the patients from day one. This is most important when dealing with vascular access. Arteriovenous fistulas (AVF), arteriovenous grafts (AVG), and permanent catheters have all been safely used as vascular access options for patients on HHD; however, an AVF is the access of choice. The most frequent adverse

Table 6-4   LETTER TO EMERGENCY MEDICAL SERVICE (EMS) AND EMERGENCY ROOM PERSONNEL

To EMS Personnel

The patient bearing this letter has end-stage kidney disease and undergoes home hemodialysis. If the patient is found connected to the hemodialysis machine and is not capable of disconnecting himself/herself, please do the following:

*INSERT SIMPLE MACHINE-SPECIFIC INSTRUCTIONS TO REMOVE PATIENT FROM MACHINE.

A diagram may be helpful

This Emergency Folder contains emergency contact information, a medical history, a medication list, and contact information for the home hemodialysis unit including on-call numbers.

Please take this documentation with you when transporting the patient to hospital.

To Emergency Room Personnel

The patient bearing this letter has end-stage kidney disease and undergoes home hemodialysis. This Emergency Folder contains emergency contact information, a medical history, a medication list, and contact information for the home hemodialysis unit including on-call numbers.

Once stabilized, please contact the home hemodialysis unit to discuss whether the current presentation is related to the home hemodialysis procedure.

Reproduced with permission from Pauly RP, Eastwood DO, Marshall MR. Patient safety in home hemodialysis: Quality assurance and serious adverse events in the home setting. *Hemodial Int.* 2015;19(Supp 1):S59-S70. Copyright © John Wiley and Sons.

events in HHD are vascular access events, particularly vascular access infections.[14] These events are certainly more common than the serious safety events listed above; however, they should not be taken lightly. Each event should be reviewed and programs should have a method for infection tracking. At minimum, tracking should include the infection type, root cause, type of vascular access involved, culture results including sensitivities, and outcome of treatment. The role of the QAI team is to help reduce the program's infection rates in part by ensuring the following:

1. The training curriculum is appropriate for each type of vascular access
2. The policies and procedures are medically appropriate and comply with infection control principles
3. Catheter reduction strategies are in place
4. Ongoing infection-related patient education is provided

Table 6-5	PROCESSES TO INITIATE AFTER A SERIOUS ADVERSE EVENT OR NEAR MISS
Step 1	Case review to determine cause and contributing circumstances of the adverse event
Step 2	Technique audit to ensure ongoing patient competence at performing home HD
Step 3	Specific questions to ask of the program: 1. Is this patient safe to continue HHD? 2. Was the adverse event avoidable? If so, how specifically? 3. Was human error the primary or a contributing factor in the adverse event? 4. Was a device defect the primary factor in the adverse event? 5. Does this event require communication with a device manufacturer (machine or disposable)? 6. Are there specific interventions required for this patient to continue home HD? 7. Is there a specific protocol or procedure that affects other HHD patients and what preventative measures should be implemented programmatically? 8. How should the information or process from question 7 be disseminated to present and future patients? 9. Does this adverse event necessitate review of the HHD recruitment or retention criteria?

HD, hemodialysis; HHD, home hemodialysis.

Reproduced with permission from Wong B, Zimmerman D, Reinties F, et al. Procedure-related serious adverse events among home hemodialysis patients: A quality assurance perspective. *Am J Kidney Dis.* 2013;63:251-258. Copyright © 2014 National Kidney Foundation, Inc. Published by Elsevier, Inc. All rights reserved. https://www.sciencedirect.com/journal/american-journal-of-kidney-diseases.

The need for ongoing education and monitoring is key because there has been a correlation identified between dialysis vintage and patient errors in vascular access-related technique possibly attributed to a false sense of invulnerability to infections, burnout, or forgetfulness concerning technique training.[14] Routine infection control audits conducted by the nurse are helpful in this area.

[For more information, see Chapters 3 and 8.]

Population-Based Clinical Outcomes

As mentioned earlier, the QAI process should include both laboratory and non-laboratory population monitoring.

Laboratory Monitoring

Percentages of patients meeting predefined laboratory goals should be reviewed and compared to internal and external benchmarks. Particular laboratory values to be monitored are discussed in the patient monitoring section. For QAI purposes, efforts to improve these outcomes should not be aimed at individual patients, but at program factors. For example, if the percentage of patients meeting the hemoglobin goal is low, the QAI team should review the effectiveness of the treatment algorithm as well as medication administration and blood collection policies. As areas needing improvement are identified, QAI projects should be initiated and outcomes measured. This is an ongoing process that should improve the quality as well as efficiency of the program.

Non-Laboratory Monitoring

Non-laboratory population monitoring is an important component of every QAI meeting and areas of focus may change based on recommendations from the program's medical director and clinical manager. For example, it may be appropriate to review the percentage of patients reaching their estimated dry weight (EDW) or percentage of patients with complete flowsheet documentation. However, certain areas should always be mentioned in order to ensure that trends are recognized and action plans implemented in a timely manner.

Vaccinations
Infection is a major cause of morbidity and mortality in the ESKD population. As previously mentioned, infection control should be reviewed with all patients and prevention strategies discussed. Vaccinations are a key component of prevention and patients should be educated accordingly. Rates of vaccination for influenza, pneumococcal pneumonia, and hepatitis B should be monitored and the IDT should work together to ensure that all medically appropriate patients consent to and feel comfortable with vaccine administration.

Vascular Access
Vascular access monitoring is an ongoing process. The QAI team should review the percentage of patients with AVFs as well as catheters.

Program-specific plans for timely access placement, access monitoring, and catheter reduction should be in place.

Transplant Listing Percentages

Transplant referrals should be made for all eligible, interested patients and the program should strive to have a majority of patients active on a transplant list. The number of patients referred, in work-up, and listed should be reviewed monthly. Each HHD facility should have information on all local transplant centers including referral criteria and required monthly testing for listed patients.

Hospitalizations

Rates and causes of hospitalizations as well as 30-day readmission rates should be reviewed by the QAI team monthly. Results should be compared to internal and external benchmarks, trends should be identified, and specific attention paid to dialysis-related hospitalizations.

Mortality

Each death should be reviewed in detail by the QAI team and each program should have a mortality-tracking tool. Serious safety events should be handled as outlined above.

▌ INDIVIDUAL PATIENT MONITORING

General Care

Although the QAI process focuses on population monitoring, it is important to remember that the population is made of individual patients. It is necessary to have national guidelines and algorithms to provide guiding principles, yet there is no substitute for individualized care.

HHD patients should be seen at least monthly by the IDT but more often depending on education and monitoring needs. At this meeting, the overall treatment plan along with non-laboratory and laboratory parameters should be reviewed. It is recommended that family members and care partners attend, ask questions, and express any concerns they may have. Their input, along with that of the patient, will help the IDT understand what is working and what areas of the treatment plan need to be adjusted.

Non-Laboratory Monitoring

Although it is easy to focus on laboratory results, non-laboratory parameters are an important aspect of HHD patient care. Areas of potential monitoring are extensive and priorities will likely change based on the patient's condition. However, there are areas that do need to be addressed each month. In fact, depending on the facility's ability to electronically transmit flowsheets, certain aspects of care may be monitored on a weekly or even daily basis. These include prescription adherence, blood pressure, weight parameters, and functionality of vascular access.

As often as possible, flowsheets should be reviewed for treatment days and times. If the patient is not performing HHD as prescribed, a root cause should be determined and the IDT should work to overcome specific barriers. Having this knowledge in a timely manner prevents worsening medical conditions and hospitalizations.

Blood pressures should be taken pre, during, and posttreatment. It is also helpful to have readings on non-HD days. Special attention should be paid to intradialytic and posttreatment hypotensive episodes. The patient should record any symptoms on the flowsheet and this information should be used to adjust medications and weight goals. Pre- and posttreatment weights should be documented, an EDW determined, and interdialytic gains calculated. As needed, changes in the patient's fluid and sodium restriction goals can be made and strategies to prevent excessive weight gains reviewed.

Vascular access is truly the patient's lifeline and should be examined at least monthly looking for any evidence of stenosis or infection. Blood flow rates as well as all difficulties in cannulation should be documented on the flowsheets. Any access issues should be addressed promptly in an attempt to maintain patency and ensure optimal dialysis treatments. Additional parameters such as vaccination rates, transplant status, QOL, and end-of-life care should be addressed by the IDT.

Laboratory Monitoring

This section will focus on frequency, types, and goals of laboratory monitoring for common sequelae of ESKD. What follows is not exhaustive but rather exemplative of the types of conditions and guidelines that are used in individual patient monitoring. It is important to remember that treatment goals change as new research emerges and guidelines are updated.

Anemia

Anemia is a common but not universal problem in HHD patients. Common causes of anemia in HD patients include erythropoietin deficiency, iron deficiency, and blood loss. The *2012 KDIGO Clinical Practice Guideline on Anemia in Chronic Kidney Disease* recommends testing for anemia every 3 months for patients on HD without anemia and defines anemia as a hemoglobin concentration less than 13 g/dL in males and less than 12 g/dL in females. For HD patients who are anemic but not currently being treated with ESAs, testing for anemia is recommended monthly. Likewise, for HD patients who are on ESA therapy, monthly hemoglobin testing is recommended both at initiation of treatment and during the maintenance phase of treatment in order to assess the success of the treatment and to adjust dosage levels of the ESA. Generally, hemoglobin levels should be monitored to maintain a level between 9 and 11.5 g/dL with some latitude to support higher levels in patients that experience improvement in their QOL. KDIGO, however, recommends avoiding levels above 13 g/dL. If laboratory monitoring reveals initial ESA hyporesponsiveness, defined as less than a 2% increase in hemoglobin concentrations after an appropriate period of time based on the amount and type of ESA used, further testing to evaluate the etiology is warranted.[15]

Iron deficiency is also a common cause of anemia in ESKD patients, and for patients with anemia iron stores should be monitored particularly if patients are on ESA therapy. Transferrin saturation and ferritin levels should be monitored at least every 3 months for patients on ESA therapy and more frequently when starting or increasing an ESA dose, when a patient has experienced blood loss, or when evaluating response to IV iron treatment. Trials of iron therapy are given when a hemoglobin rise or ESA dose reduction is desired, the transferrin saturation levels are less than or equal to 30%, and the ferritin levels are less than or equal to 500 ng/mL.

Mineral and Bone Disorder

Mineral and bone disorder (MBD) in ESKD comprises several interrelated disorders including abnormal calcium and phosphorous metabolism, secondary hyperparathyroidism (HPT), and vitamin D deficiency. The *2017 KDIGO Clinical Practice Guideline Update for the Diagnosis, Evaluation, and Treatment of Chronic Kidney Disease—Mineral and Bone Disorder* advocates basing the frequency of monitoring of calcium, phosphate, and parathyroid hormone (PTH) on the presence and magnitude of the abnormalities and the rate of progression of the underlying chronic kidney disease (CKD).[16] For those on HD, the guidelines recommend checking serum calcium and phosphorous every 1 to 3 months, PTH levels every 3 to 6 months, and alkaline phosphatase actively at least every 12 months or more frequently if PTH is elevated. The guideline also recommends measuring 25-hydroxyvitamin D (calcidiol) levels and then determining the frequency of testing based on baseline values and whether treatment is needed. Initiation and goals of therapy will be dependent on the normal ranges of the laboratory parameters. The guideline also suggests that HD patients with MBD and/or risk factors for osteoporosis undergo bone mineral density testing to assess fracture risk if the results will impact treatment decisions. Likewise, the guideline suggests that for those patients for whom the type of renal osteodystrophy will impact treatment decisions, bone marrow biopsy may also be reasonable.

Acid/Base

Metabolic acidosis is common among HHD patients, stemming from decreased ability to excrete volatile acids produced in the course of normal metabolism. The inability to excrete acid leads to a depletion of the body's bicarbonate buffering system that is replenished in part through the dialysis procedure. The *2000 NKF KDOQI Nutrition in Chronic Renal Failure Guidelines* recommend monitoring serum bicarbonate in maintenance dialysis patients monthly and maintaining levels at or above 22 mmol/L.[17]

Electrolytes

Electrolyte abnormalities, namely potassium, magnesium, and sodium disorders, are common in dialysis patients and are associated with increased morbidity and mortality. Therefore, electrolytes should be monitored frequently and corrected as needed in all HHD patients.

Nutrition

Malnutrition is a common comorbidity in dialysis patients. The *2000 KDOQI Nutrition in Chronic Renal Failure* guidelines recommend periodic assessment of a combination of complementary measures including serum albumin, percent of usual body weight, percent of standard body weight, subjective assessments, dietary interviews, and normalized protein nitrogen appearance.[17]

Diabetes

Diabetes mellitus is the leading cause of ESKD in the United States and is associated with increased risk of significant cardiovascular comorbidity. *The American Diabetes Association 2018 Standards of Medical Care* recommends hemoglobin A1C monitoring at least biannually in diabetic patients with stable glycemic control and quarterly in patients who are not meeting glycemic goals or in whom therapy has changed.[18]

Hepatitis C

Hepatitis C is a common and significant comorbidity in HD patients that increases the risk of liver failure and development of hepatocellular carcinoma.[19] Effective treatment regimens are available for patients on HD. The *2018 KDIGO Clinical Practice Guideline for the Prevention, Diagnosis, Evaluation, and Treatment of Hepatitis C in Chronic Kidney Disease* recommends screening all patients for the hepatitis C virus (HCV) when they initiate HHD and when they transfer from another dialysis facility or modality.[20] Patients should also be screened during kidney transplantation evaluations. Given the risk of transmission for in-center dialysis patients, follow-up HCV screening is recommended every 6 months. The guideline also recommends checking alanine aminotransferase (ALT) levels upon initiation of in-center HD or upon transfer from other facilities and at monthly intervals. HHD patients that are transferred in-center should also follow these guidelines. For patients with both CKD and HCV, periodic liver testing is suggested as well as screening for hepatitis A, hepatitis B, and human immunodeficiency virus (HIV).

Adequacy

Adequate dialysis is a multifocal concept including both solute and fluid removal, yet the term "adequacy" is often used to refer to solute clearance alone. Solute clearance is typically expressed as Kt/V, where K_{urea} is the effective (delivered) dialyzer urea clearance in milliliters per minute integrated over the entire dialysis session, t_d is the time in minutes measured from beginning to end of dialysis, and V_{urea} is the patient's volume of urea distribution in milliliters. The *KDOQI Clinical Practice Guideline for Hemodialysis Adequacy: 2015 Update* recommends for those patients dialyzing more than three times per week aiming for a standard Kt/V of 2.3 volumes per week with a minimum delivered dose of 2.1 using a method of calculation that includes the contribution of ultrafiltration (UF) and residual renal function (RRF). We recommend monitoring at Kt/V at least monthly.[21]

▌CONCLUSION

The principles of monitoring and healthcare-related quality are the basis for an effective and safe HHD program. In this chapter, we discussed how these principles should be applied to both population-based QAI and individual patient care. Although these are indeed separate components and should be approached differently, they are very much related. As the QAI team works to improve the program's QAI process and efficiency, it creates an environment in which individual patients can thrive, and when individual patients do well, the population as a whole succeeds.

▌REFERENCES

1. Understanding Quality Measurement. Content last reviewed October 2018. Agency for Healthcare Research and Quality, Rockville, MD. Available at https://www.ahrq.gov/professionals/quality-patient-safety/quality-resources/tools/chtoolbx/understand/index.html. Accessed November 7, 2019.
2. The National Forum of ESRD Networks. Available at https://esrdnetworks.org/resources/toolkits. Accessed November 7, 2019.
3. Abrahim A, Chan CT. Managing kidney failure with home hemodialysis. *Clin J Am Soc Nephrol*. 2019;14:1268-1273.
4. Department of Health and Human Services. Centers for Medicare & Medicaid Services: Quality, safety & oversight—guidance to laws & regulations—dialysis. Available at https://www.cms.gov/Medicare/Provider-Enrollment-and-Certification/GuidanceforLawsAndRegulations/Dialysis.html. Accessed November 7, 2019.
5. Department of Health and Human Services. Centers for Medicare & Medicaid Services: ESRD Surveyor Training Interpretive Guidance Final Version 1.1. Available at https://www.cms.gov/Medicare/Provider-Enrollment-and-Certification/GuidanceforLawsAndRegulations/Downloads/esrdpgmguidance.pdf. Accessed November 7, 2019.
6. Moran J, Kraus M. Starting a home hemodialysis program. *Semin Dial*. 2007;20(1):35-39.
7. Nesrallah GE, Lindsay RM, Cuerden MS, et al. Intensive hemodialysis associates with improved survival compared with conventional hemodialysis. *J Am Soc Nephrol*. 2012;23:696-705.
8. Juergensen E, Wuerth D, Finkelstein SH, Juergensen PH, Bekuli A, Finkelstein FO. Hemodialysis and peritoneal dialysis: patients' assessment of their satisfaction with therapy and the impact of the therapy on their lives. *Clin J Am Soc Nephrol*. 2006;1:1191-1196.
9. Gilbertson EL, Krishnasamy R, Foote C, Kennard AL, Jardine MJ, Gray NA. Burden of care and quality of life among caregivers for adults receiving maintenance dialysis: a systemic review. *Am J Kidney Dis*. 2019;73:332-343.
10. Marshall MR, Chan CT, eds. *Implementing Hemodialysis in the Home: A Practical Manual*. Indianapolis, IN: International Society of Hemodialysis; 2016.
11. Centers for Medicare & Medicaid Services. *Preparing for Emergencies: A Guide for People on Dialysis*. 2nd ed. Baltimore, MD: Centers for Medicare & Medicaid Services; 2017.
12. Wong B, Zimmerman D, Reinties F, et al. Procedure-related serious adverse events among home hemodialysis patients: a quality assurance perspective. *Am J Kidney Dis*. 2013;63:251-258.
13. Pauly RP, Eastwood DO, Marshall MR. Patient safety in home hemodialysis: quality assurance and serious adverse events in the home setting. *Hemodial Int*. 2015;19(suppl 1):S59-S70.
14. Rousseau-Gagnon M, Faratro R, D'Gama C, et al. The use of vascular access audit and infections in home hemodialysis. *Hemodial Int*. 2016;20(2):298-305.

15. Kidney Disease: Improving Global Outcomes (KDIGO) Anemia Work Group. KDIGO clinical practice guideline for anemia in chronic kidney disease. *Kidney Int Suppl.* 2012;2:279-335.

16. Kidney Disease: Improving Global Outcomes (KDIGO) CKD-MBD Update Work Group. KDIGO 2017 clinical practice guideline update for the diagnosis, evaluation, prevention, and treatment of chronic kidney disease–mineral and bone disorder (CKD-MBD). *Kidney Int Suppl.* 2017;7:1-59.

17. K/DOQI, National Kidney Foundation. Clinical practice guidelines for nutrition in chronic renal failure. *Am J Kidney Dis.* 2000;35(6 suppl 2):S1-S140.

18. American Diabetes Association. 6. Glycemic targets: standards of medical care in diabetes—2018. *Diabetes Care.* 2018;41(suppl 1):S55-S64.

19. Simonetti RG, Camma C, Fiorello F, et al. Hepatitis C virus infection as a risk factor for hepatocellular carcinoma in patients with cirrhosis: a case-control study. *Ann Intern Med.* 1992;116(2):97-102.

20. Kidney Disease: Improving Global Outcomes (KDIGO) Hepatitis C Work Group. KDIGO 2018 clinical practice guideline for the prevention, diagnosis, evaluation, and treatment of hepatitis C in chronic kidney disease. *Kidney Int Suppl.* 2018;8:91-165.

21. K/DOQI, National Kidney Foundation. Clinical practice guideline for hemodialysis adequacy: 2015 update. *Am J Kidney Dis.* 2015;66(5):884-930.

7

OVERVIEW OF BENEFITS AND LIMITATIONS OF HOME HEMODIALYSIS

Alice Chedid and Daphne H. Knicely

❚ CARDIOVASCULAR DISEASE

Despite the advances in the management of end-stage kidney disease (ESKD) in recent years, cardiovascular disease remains the leading cause of death in ESKD patients and the principal discharge diagnosis accompanying one in four hospital admissions.[1] In addition to traditional cardiovascular risk factors, dialysis patients have additional risks, including ongoing exposure to volume overload, hyperphosphatemia, chronic inflammation, and uremic toxins. These risk factors can contribute to impaired structure and function of the heart and promote further progression of cardiovascular disease.[2]

[For more information, see Chapter 9.]

Left Ventricular Mass

An important predictor of cardiovascular morbidity and mortality in dialysis patients is left ventricular hypertrophy (LVH). In new dialysis patients, the prevalence of LVH is as high as 75%. Given that left ventricular mass (LVM) is an independent predictor of cardiovascular mortality, regression of LVH may reduce overall cardiovascular risk. Intensive hemodialysis (HD) has been shown to reduce LVM in multiple randomized trials. For example, the Frequent Hemodialysis Network (FHN) trial showed that short daily and nocturnal HD schedules were associated with significant reduction in the mean LVM from 142 g to 125 g (a 12% decrease), while decreasing only modestly with the conventional thrice-weekly HD schedule from 141 g to 138 g.

In a randomized controlled trial conducted at two Canadian institutions between August 2004 and December 2006, a total of 52 patients were recruited. The primary outcome was to compare the effects of frequent nocturnal hemodialysis (NHD) versus conventional hemodialysis (CHD) on change in LVM. The LVM decreased by a mean (SD) of 13.8 (23.0) g in the NHD group and increased by 1.5 (24.0) g in the CHD group ($P=0.04$).[2]

[For more information, see Chapter 9.]

Blood Pressure

Hypertension is very common in dialysis patients and may often be poorly controlled. Sodium and volume overload are the prominent mechanisms contributing to high blood pressure. Other mechanisms include arterial stiffness, activation of renin-angiotensin-aldosterone and sympathetic nervous systems, endothelial dysfunction, and sleep apnea. Multiple pharmacological and non-pharmacological interventions including increasing frequency of dialysis have been implemented in this population.[3]

In 1999, Woods et al. evaluated 72 patients that started daily HD between 1972 and 1996. Their predialysis systolic and diastolic blood pressures fell by 7 and 4 mm Hg respectively, after starting frequent HD

(P=0.02). There was a statistically significant reduction in the number of antihypertensive medications prescribed during the 12 months after switching to daily HD. The percentage of patients receiving no antihypertensive medications increased from 54% to 61% at 6 months and 75% at 12 months after the switch to daily HD. The fraction of patients receiving more than one antihypertensive medication also decreased.[4]

More recently, in 2009, David et al. showed that more intensified nocturnal HD was associated with a decrease in predialytic mean arterial pressure (MAP) (100 vs. 89 mm Hg) and postdialytic MAP (97 vs. 83 mm Hg) after a period of 1 year. This improvement in blood pressure occurred despite a reduction in the use of antihypertensive medications.[5]

[For more information, see Chapter 9.]

ANEMIA AND ERYTHROPOIESIS-STIMULATING AGENT USE

Anemia, which is defined as a hemoglobin <12 g/dL, is a common complication in ESKD, affecting approximately 75% of patients. Although the cause of anemia is multifactorial, the main cause is deficiency in the production of erythropoietin by the kidneys, which can be treated by administering erythropoiesis-stimulating agents (ESAs).[6] However, hyporesponsiveness to ESAs is not uncommon and one known mechanism is the delivery of inadequate dialysis.[7]

Klarenbach et al. conducted a 3-year prospective observational study of patients who received "daily" HD (daily short high-efficiency home HD or long slow nocturnal HD) and CHD. The mean erythropoietin dose fell in the "daily" group from 87 to 53 U/week/kg (P=0.020). The mean hemoglobin rose from 11.5 ($\pm$1.8) to 12.9 ($\pm$1.4) g/dL (P=0.008). There was no significant change in erythropoietin dose or hemoglobin in the CHD group.[7] Another study from Ornt et al. examined the effects of ESA dosing and hemoglobin concentrations with more frequent HD. The study looked at subjects enrolled in the FHN daily and nocturnal trials. It showed no significant treatment effect in the six times versus three times per week treatment groups on logESA dose or the ratio of log of ESA dose to hemoglobin concentration. They concluded that more frequent HD did not have a significant or clinically important effect on anemia management.[8]

In 2015, Poon et al. in Hong Kong published a retrospective controlled study investigating whether anemia and ESA requirements improved in patients receiving every other day nocturnal home hemodialysis (HHD) (23 patients) compared with CHD (25 patients). At 24 months, hemoglobin level increased by 1.98 ($\pm$2.74) g/dL in the nocturnal HHD group while it decreased by 0.20 ($\pm$2.32) g/dL in the CHD group (P=0.007). ESA requirements decreased by 53.49 ($\pm$55.50) U/kg/week in the nocturnal HHD patients whereas it increased by 16.22 ($\pm$ 50.01) U/kg/week in the CHD group (P < 0.001). Twenty-six percent of nocturnal HHD patients were able to discontinue ESA use compared with none in the CHD group.[9]

▌MINERAL BONE METABOLISM

Phosphate Control

Abnormalities in mineral bone metabolism have contributed to all-cause and cardiovascular mortality in ESKD. Despite rigorous efforts by nephrologists to counsel patients about the importance of mineral bone disease, hyperphosphatemia remains a significant problem among patients receiving CHD. CHD does not remove sufficient phosphate. A 4-hour HD session will clear 34 mmol of phosphate (1054 mg of phosphorus), which is not sufficient to keep up with the typical phosphorus intake of 800 to 2000 mg/day (equivalent to 25.8 to 64.5 mmol of phosphate) in the Western diet.[10]

Given the above, there has been increasing interest in daily dialysis to improve phosphate control. Ayus et al. analyzed data from a 12-month, prospective, non-randomized, controlled study of daily HD versus CHD. They particularly focused on phosphate control. The mean serum phosphorus was significantly lower in the daily HD subjects than in the CHD subjects at 12-month follow-up (4.20 vs. 5.02 mg/dL, P=0.0001). In addition, the percentage of subjects using phosphate binders decreased from 77% to 40% (P=0.01) in the daily HD group and did not change in the CHD group.[11]

[For more information, see Chapter 10.]

▌INFLAMMATION

Chronic inflammation is an independent risk factor for cardiovascular death in ESKD. Causes of chronic inflammation may include dialyzer incompatibility, acidosis, oxidative stress, dialysate contamination, and occult infection of clotted arteriovenous grafts (AVG). Few therapeutic options are available for dialysis patients to reduce inflammatory markers—short daily HD may be an effective intervention.[12] Ayus et al. also examined the effects of short daily hemodialysis (SDHD) on inflammation compared to CHD. At baseline, there was no difference in the C-reactive protein levels between the two groups. In patients who underwent SDHD, there was a decrease in median C-reactive protein levels between baseline and at 6 and 12 months ($P < 0.01$) with a 95% reduction at 12 months. In addition, the percentage of patients with normal C-reactive protein levels increased from 19% to 61% ($P=0.006$) between the start of the study and the end of follow-up.[11]

▌ NUTRITIONAL STATUS

Malnutrition is a common problem and is associated with increased morbidity and mortality in ESKD. Malnutrition is thought to be multifactorial, due to accumulation of uremic toxins, low protein energy intake, and metabolic hormonal abnormalities.[13] Galland et al. showed that more frequent HD was associated with better nutritional markers in a French population. The improvement in nutritional status was attributed to improved sense of well-being and resulting improvement in appetite and increased food intake. An alternative explanation was better clearance of anorexic factors with daily HD. The average daily intake of protein, carbohydrates, and lipids increased at 6 and 12 months after switching to more frequent HD. Serum albumin, prealbumin, and total cholesterol level increased at 6 and 12 months after switching to daily HD. These changes were accompanied by increase in dry body weight and lean body mass.[13] Ayus et al. analyzed nutritional markers as a secondary outcome. In the daily HD group, there was significant increase in normalized protein catabolic rate from baseline to the end of the study, compared to no change in the CHD group.[11]

▌ FERTILITY

Dialysis patients have a lower conception rate and worse pregnancy outcomes compared to non-dialysis patients. Infertility is more common and may be secondary to endocrine abnormalities including decreased prolactin clearance, lower levels of estrogen and progesterone, and higher but constant levels of luteinizing hormone. All of these abnormalities can lead to dysregulation of the pituitary-hypothalamic axis that may ultimately result in infertility. Although published data remains scarce, it is well established that intensive HD regimens improve fertility in ESKD patients. Increased toxin clearance may partially restore the pituitary-hypothalamic axis, decrease high prolactin levels, and increase testosterone levels.[14] Eps et al. followed 30 men and 7 women in Australia who converted from CHD to every other day nocturnal HHD. In men, there

was a significant improvement in hyperprolactinemia and hypotestostero-
nemia. One male patient successfully fathered a child without the assistance of any fertility method. He had been unsuccessful for many years
while on CHD. Among the women, two out of the three women who were
less than 40 years old had return of regular menses.[15]

EXERCISE CAPACITY

Exercise capacity, which is assessed by peak oxygen uptake (VO_2 peak),
is reduced by 40% in ESKD patients. The reasons for this may include
anemia, impaired muscle perfusion, reduced muscle mass, and associated
comorbid conditions. Chan et al. followed 12 HD patients, who were transitioned from CHD to a more intense HD regimen. The exercise duration increased progressively as well as the exercise capacity at 2, 3, and 6
months. The authors concluded that the augmented uremia control with
more intense HD improved both exercise capacity and duration.[16]

SLEEP AND RESTLESS LEG SYNDROME

Poor sleep quality is a common symptom among patients receiving CHD,
with 41% to 83% patients reporting insomnia, sleep disordered breathing,
and excessive daytime sleepiness. The prevalence of restless leg syndrome
(RLS) is also high among patients receiving CHD, with estimates ranging
between 6% and 62%.[17] Patients with RLS suffer from sleep fragmenta-
tion, sleep deprivation, anxiety, and depressive symptoms.

The Following Rehabilitation, Economics and Everyday-Dialysis
Outcome Measurements (FREEDOM) study investigated the benefits of
home SDHD. They looked at the long-term effect of SDHD on the prevalence and severity of RLS, and prevalence of sleep disturbances. One
hundred twenty-seven out of 235 participants completed the 12-month
follow up. There was a decline in the percentage of patients reporting RLS
symptoms from 35% to 26% and of those reporting RLS symptoms as
moderate-to-severe RLS (59% to 43%). The results for the sleep survey
were similar. There was improvement in several scales even after adjusting
for presence of RLS and the use of anxiolytics and hypnotics.[17]

DEPRESSION AND POSTDIALYSIS RECOVERY TIME

The FREEDOM study also examined the long-term impact of daily HD
on depressive symptoms and postdialysis recovery time. The investigators

used the Beck Depression Inventory (BDI) survey and a previously vali- dated questionnaire for postdialysis recovery time. The BDI survey and postdialysis recovery time questionnaire were administered at baseline, and changes were assessed at 4 and 12 months. One hundred twenty-eight patients out of 239 completed the study. There was a significant decrease in mean BDI score over 12 months (11.2 vs. 7.8; $P < 0.001$). Also, the percentage of patients with depressive symptoms (BDI score >10) signifi- cantly decreased over 12 months (41% vs. 27%; $P=0.03$). Similarly, there was a significant decrease in postdialysis recovery time over 12 months (476 vs. 63 minutes; $P < 0.001$). The percentage of patients experienc- ing prolonged postdialysis recovery time (≥60 minutes) also significantly decreased (81% vs. 35%; $P=0.001$).[18]

▌QUALITY OF LIFE

While the definition of quality of care is broad, health-related quality of life (Hr-QOL) is easily defined. It encompasses the mental and physi- cal health of patients and their consequences. Hr-QOL is assessed using questionnaires—good communication is important.[19] Many observa- tional studies have shown that daily HD improves quality of life (QOL). In the study by Culleton et al., QOL was examined as a secondary out- come. There was no difference in the QOL between patients on CHD and patients on frequent NHD. The scores appeared to deteriorate over time in both groups. However, there was statistically significant improvements within the frequent NHD group in selected kidney-specific domains of QOL including effects and burden of kidney disease.[2]

[For more information, see Chapter 11.]

▌HOSPITALIZATION

As discussed previously in this chapter, it is known that HHD improves some parameters of cardiovascular function. Weinhandl et al. investigated whether daily HHD was associated with lower hospitalization risk. In 3480 daily HHD and 17,400 thrice-weekly in-center HD patients enrolled in the study, there was no difference in all-cause admission for daily HHD versus in-center HD, but there were fewer admissions for cardiovascular disease (hazard ratio 0.89, 0.86 to 0.93).[20]

In a subsequent study, Weinhandl et al. compared hospitalization rates in daily HHD versus peritoneal dialysis (PD) patients in a matched cohort study. They matched 4201 new HHD patients from 2007 to 2010 with 4201 new PD patients from the US Renal Data System (USRDS) database. HHD was associated with an 8% lower risk for all-cause hospitalization (hazard ratio 0.92, 0.89 to 0.95). However, HHD patients had a higher rate of admission secondary to infection, with a hazard ratio of 1.18 (1.13 to 1.23). The principal diagnoses were bacteremia/sepsis, cardiac infection, osteomyelitis, and vascular access infection.[21]

[For more information, see Chapter 12.]

PERCEIVED BENEFITS

Pipkin et al. conducted a survey to identify the benefits of HHD as perceived by patients on conventional in-center HD.[22] Over 66 of respondents identified the following incentives for considering switching to HHD: flexible scheduling and prescription, less travel to dialysis units, more liberal diet, partner encouragement, influence of other home dialysis patients, more privacy, and putative improvement in well-being.

PERCEIVED LIMITATIONS

Pipkin and colleagues found that the two most common barriers preventing in-center HD patients from considering a switch to HHD were lack of motivation and patients being very comfortable with in-center HD and not being willing to make any changes.[22] Other barriers noted by 66% of respondents included fear of self-cannulation, fear of needles, fear of inability to sleep during treatment, high level of comorbid disease, lack of family/partner support, fear of the machine, and fear of inability to learn the machine.

TRAINING

HHD training involves significant commitment of time and energy by the patient and care partner. Typically, training requires 4 to 6 weeks. In an analysis of HHD training duration, Pipkin found that the mean number of HHD training sessions was 27.7 ($\pm$10.4) days. The average training time for patients using a catheter was marginally less than patients using an arteriovenous fistula (AVF). Patients who had experience in a self-care center also required fewer training sessions. Education level had no impact on training time. There was no difference in the number of training sessions for those who did not have education beyond high school compared with those who did ($P = 0.72$).[21] Age was positively associated with training time. On average, three additional training sessions were required for each decade increase in age. In addition to age, the number of comorbidities also correlated with training time. Patients with a higher modified Charlson comorbidity score required more training.[21]

HOME ENVIRONMENT

HHD requires an adequate home environment. The room where the HHD machine will be located should be well lighted, comfortable, and easy to clean.[23] Some renovations, such as electrical upgrades and plumbing modifications, may be required to make the home suitable for HHD. If the water treatment system uses reverse osmosis, equipment that increases water pressure and ensures appropriate water temperatures may need to be installed.[23]

PARTNER REQUIREMENT

For HHD there is usually a requirement for a care partner. Given that HD patients are commonly older and have multiple comorbidities, it is understandable to require the presence of a partner. The partner often assists in or performs the setup, takedown, and cleaning of the machine. There is concern for care partner burnout and workload particularly in HHD patients given the increase in dialysis frequency and duration.[23]

Rioux et al. evaluated care partner burden among nocturnal HHD patients in Ontario, Canada. Cross-sectional surveys were sent to 61 established nocturnal HHD patients and their care partners. Compared to care partners, patients had lower perceived physical health scores but had similar mental health scores. Depression criteria were present in 47% of patients and 25% of care partners. Although the total global burden perceived by either care partners or patients is relatively low, a significant proportion of both groups fulfilled criteria for depression.[24]

[For more information, see Chapters 2 and 11.]

VASCULAR ACCESS

The most common cannulation techniques for an AVF are buttonhole and rope-ladder. In buttonhole cannulation, a needle is inserted in the same spot, at the same angle, at the same depth, every time, eventually creating a tract that can be cannulated with a blunt needle. This type of cannulation has gained popularity in HHD. The rope-ladder cannulation involves rotating the cannulation sites up and down the length of the access.[25]

[For more information, see Chapters 3 and 8.]

Table 7-1 SUMMARY OF ADVANTAGES AND CHALLENGES OF HOME HEMODIALYSIS	
Summary	
Advantages of Home Hemodialysis	**Challenges Associated with Home Hemodialysis**
• Improved LVM • Better blood pressure control and reduction in antihypertensive medications • Improvement in anemia, increased responsiveness to ESAs, and reduction in ESA dosing • Improved serum phosphate values and reduction in phosphorus binder use • Reduction in markers of chronic inflammation • Enhanced nutritional status as evidenced by improved nutritional markers • Improvement in sex hormone levels in both males and females • Improved exercise duration and capacity • Improvement in prevalence and severity of RLS symptoms • Improved sleep quality • Improvement in depressive symptoms • Reduction in postdialysis recovery time • Improvement in selected kidney-specific QOL parameters • Reduction in hospitalization	• Lack of motivation to perform home hemodialysis • Increasing age and comorbidities that deter home hemodialysis • Fear of self-cannulation and needles • Lack of family/partner support • Fear of complications related to home hemodialysis and lack of healthcare team support • Need for home renovations to support home hemodialysis • Increased vascular access infections and interventions

ESA, erythropoiesis-stimulating agent; LVM, left ventricular mass; QOL, quality of life; RLS, restless leg syndrome.

Infections

A prospective study by Lok et al. examined 631 patients who were dialyzed using an AVF from 2001 to 2010 in Toronto and Ottawa. The rate of buttonhole-related infections was high among patients on frequent HD and more than 50 times greater than that among patients on conventional in-center HD using the rope-ladder technique. There were 39 episodes of buttonhole-related bacteremia (85% caused by *S. aureus*) and at least 2 local buttonhole site infections. There were five (13%) infection-related hospitalizations and three (10%) serious metastatic infections, including fistula loss. In comparison, there was one possible fistula-related infection in the conventional in-center HD group during follow-up.[26]

[For more information, see Chapter 3.]

Access Interventions

Given the increase in frequency of dialysis, multiple studies have showed increase in vascular access interventions in patients on HHD compared to CHD. In 2010, the FHN group published a randomized controlled trial that analyzed the difference between in-center HD six times per week versus three times per week. Patients who underwent more dialysis were more likely to undergo vascular access interventions. There were 95 interventions related to vascular access (19 interventions to correct access failure and 76 other procedures) in the frequent HD group and 65 interventions (23 to correct access failure and 42 other procedures) in the CHD group.[27]

In Australia, Jun et al. looked at the outcomes of extended hours on HD performed at home. They looked at patients from six different centers, total of 286 patients. Higher dialysis frequency was associated with a higher risk to developing an access event. The hazard ratio per dialysis session was 1.56 (1.03 to 2.36). The access events included infection, thrombosis/occlusion, AVF aneurysm, stenosis, and AVF revision requirement. The rate of access infection was particularly high, affecting 59.5% of patients. The access-related events were a significant predictor of death (hazard ratio 2.85; 1.14 to 7.15; $P=0.03$). Given this, there was a concern that access events will negatively affect long-term outcomes.[28]

[For more information, see Chapter 3.]

In summary, HHD is a modality of kidney replacement therapy that has been shown to be beneficial to ESKD patients. It is generally safe and requires patients to be involved in their own care with an anticipation of significant improvements in health outcomes and resource utilization[23] (Table 7-1).

▌REFERENCES

1. McCullough P, Chan C, Weinhandl E, Burkart J, Bakris G. Intensive hemodialysis, left ventricular hypertrophy, and cardiovascular disease. *Am J Kidney Dis.* 2016;68(5S1):S5-S14.

2. Culleton B, Walsh M, Klarenbach S, et al. Effect of frequent nocturnal hemodialysis vs conventional hemodialysis on left ventricular mass and quality of life. *JAMA.* 2007;298(11):1291-1299.

3. Sarafidis P, Persu A, Agarwal R, et al. Hypertension in dialysis patients: a consensus document by the European Renal and Cardiovascular Medicine

(EURECA-m) working group of the European Renal Association—European Dialysis and Transplant Association (ERA-EDTA) and the Hypertension and the Kidney working group of the European Society of Hypertension. *J Hypertens.* 2017;35(4):657-676.

4. Woods J, Port F, Orzol S, et al. Clinical and biochemical correlates of starting "daily" hemodialysis. *Kidney Int.* 1999; 55:2467-2476.

5. David S, Kumpers P, Eisenbach G, Haller H, Kielstein JT. Prospective evaluation of an in-center conversion from conventional hemodialysis to an intensified nocturnal strategy. *Nephrol Dial Transplant.* 2009;24(7):2232-2240.

6. Johnson D, Pascoe E, Badve S, et al. A randomized, placebo-controlled trial of pentoxifylline on erythropoiesis-stimulating agent hyporesponsiveness in anemic patients with CKD: the Handling Erythropoietin Resistance with Oxpentifylline (HERO) trial. *Am J Kidney Dis.* 2015;65(1):49-57.

7. Klarenbach S, Heidenheim P, Leitch R, Lindsay, Daily/Nocturnal Dialysis Study Group. Reduced requirement for erythropoietin with quotidian hemodialysis therapy. *ASAIO J.* 2002;48:57-61.

8. Ornt DB, Larive B, Rastogi A, et al. Impact of frequent hemodialysis on anemia management: results from the Frequent Hemodialysis Network (FHN) trials. *Nephrol Dial Transplant.* 2013;28(7):1888-1898.

9. Poon C, Tang H, Wong J, et al. Effect of alternate night nocturnal home hemodialysis on anemia control in patients with end-stage renal disease. *Hemodial Int.* 2015;19:235-241.

10. Achinger S, Ayus J. The role of daily dialysis in the control of hyperphosphatemia. *Kidney Int.* 2005;67(S95):S28-S32.

11. Ayus J, Achinger S, Mizani M, et al. Phosphorus balance and mineral metabolism with 3h daily hemodialysis. *Kidney Int.* 2007;71(4):336-342.

12. Ayus J, Mizani M, Achinger S, Thadhani R, Go AS, Lee S. Effects of short daily versus conventional hemodialysis on left ventricular hypertrophy and inflammatory markers: a prospective, controlled study. *J Am Soc Nephrol.* 2005;16(9):2778-2788.

13. Galland R, Traeger J. Short daily hemodialysis and nutritional status in patients with chronic renal failure. *Semin Dial.* 2004;17(2):104-108.

14. Tennankore K, Nadeau-Fredette A, Chan C. Intensified home hemodialysis: clinical benefits, risks and target populations. *Nephrol Dial Transplant.* 2014;29(7):1342-1349.

15. Eps C, Hawley C, Jeffries J, et al. Changes in serum prolactin, sex hormones and thyroid function with alternate nightly nocturnal home haemodialysis. *Nephrology (Carlton).* 2012;17(1):42-47.

16. Chan C, Notarius C, Merlocco A, Floras JS. Improvement in exercise duration and capacity after conversion to nocturnal home haemodialysis. *Nephrol Dial Transplant.* 2007;22(11):3285-3291.

17. Jaber B, Schiller B, Burkart J, et al. Impact of short daily hemodialysis on restless legs symptoms and sleep disturbances. *Clin J Am Soc Nephrol.* 2011;6(5):1049-1056.

18. Jaber B, Lee Y, Collins A, et al. Effect of daily hemodialysis on depressive symptoms and post-dialysis recovery time: interim report from the FREEDOM (Following Rehabilitation, Economics and Everyday-Dialysis Outcome Measurements) study. *Am J Kidney Dis.* 2010;56(3):531-539.

19. Mooney A. Quality of life: questionnaires and questions. *J Health Commun.* 2006;11(3):327-341.

20. Weinhandl E, Nieman K, Gilbertson D, Collins AJ. Hospitalization in daily home hemodialysis and matched thrice-weekly in-center hemodialysis patients. *Am J Kidney Dis.* 2015;65(1):98-108.

21. Weinhandl E, Gilbertson D, Collins AJ. Mortality, hospitalizations and technique failure in daily home hemodialysis and matched peritoneal dialysis patients: a matched cohort study. *Am J Kidney Dis.* 2016;67(1):98-110.

22. Pipkin M, Eggers PW, Larive B, et al. Recruitment and training for home hemodialysis: experience and lessons from the nocturnal dialysis trial. *Clin J Am Soc Nephrol.* 2010;5:1614-1620.

23. Karkar A, Hegbrant J, Strippoli G. Benefits and implementation of home hemodialysis: a narrative review. *Saudi J Kidney Dis Transpl.* 2015;26(6):1095-1107.

24. Rioux J, Narayanan R, Chan C. Caregiver burden among nocturnal home hemodialysis patients. *Hemodial Int.* 2012;16(2):214-219.

25. Hawley C, Jeffries J, Nearhos J, Eps CV. Complications of home hemodialysis. *Hemodial Int.* 2008;12:S21-S25.

26. Lok C, Sontrop J, Faratro R, Chan C, Zimmerman DL. Frequent hemodialysis fistula infectious complications. *Nephron Extra.* 2014;4(3):159-167.

27. The FHN Trial Group. In-center hemodialysis six times per week versus three times per week. *N Engl J Med.* 2010;363(4):2287-2300.

28. Jun M, Jardine M, Gray N, et al. Outcomes of extended-hours hemodialysis performed predominantly at home. *Am J Kidney Dis.* 2013;61(2):247-253.

COMPLICATIONS OF HOME HEMODIALYSIS

8

Tushar Chopra, Lakshmi Kannan,
and Emaad M. Abdel-Rahman

The crude prevalence of end-stage kidney disease (ESKD) is 2160.7 per million in the United States, with only 2% of these patients utilizing home hemodialysis (HHD).[1] The number of HHD patients has increased in recent years and is expected to increase further following the introduction of the United States Department of Health and Human Services Advancing American Kidney Health Initiative. While HHD has been associated with multiple benefits,[2–7] it is not without complications. Nephrologists must be knowledgeable about these complications as HHD use increases in the United States. In this chapter, we discuss technical, medical, and psychosocial complications associated with HHD and their diagnosis, management, and prevention.

GENERAL CONSIDERATIONS

The HHD room setup is quite important. In order to minimize the risk of complications, all screens for devices should be in direct line of sight with adequate lighting. The space utilized for HHD should have low humidity, a comfortable temperature, telephone access, and restricted access to children and pets. Availability of easy-to-use sinks with hands-free elbow taps would be ideal. All surfaces and furnishings should be easy to clean.

TECHNICAL COMPLICATIONS

The summary of technical complications is provided in Table 8-1.

Hemorrhage

Bleeding is an uncommon but serious complication of HHD. In two studies evaluating adverse events in HHD programs in Canada, blood loss was the most common life-threatening adverse effect.[8,9] Bleeding can occur in three areas: at the access through needle dislodgment or disconnection from a catheter, from the dialysis circuit, or into the dialysis circuit. Needle dislodgement (venous port disconnection) was the leading cause of hemorrhage in these studies, mostly due to patients using incorrect cannulation or taping technique.[8] Hemorrhage following venous port disconnection can occur if the change in venous pressure is not significant enough to cause the machine to alarm and the pump to stop. If venous dislodgement is not promptly identified and the pump turned off, significant blood loss and death can occur.

Several measures can be utilized to avoid fatal hemorrhage, including increased vigilance from both the patient and the care partner. Needles should be firmly secured to avoid dislodgement. The dialysis access and tubing should remain visible throughout the dialysis treatment. Disconnecting the arterial needle before the venous needle may decrease the risk of bleeding. Use of blood leak detectors should be considered. One study in a small cohort of HHD patients in Canada examined the use of blood leak detectors and venous line clamps that are activated when

Table 8-1 TECHNICAL COMPLICATIONS	
Problem	**Solution**
Hemorrhage	
At the access	Stop blood pump and apply direct pressure on access
	Preventive measures
	• Secure needles at the insertion site
	• Keep dialysis access and tubing visible throughout the treatment
	• Use blood leak detectors
	• Disconnect the arterial needle before the venous needle
From the dialysis circuit	Keep dialysis access and tubing visible throughout treatment
	Stop blood pump
Into the dialysis circuit	Heed blood leak alarm
	Stop blood pump
Air embolism	
Between access and blood pump	Heed air detection alarms
	Clamp venous line
	Stop the blood pump
	Place patient supine
	Call local emergency medical personnel
During connection	Heed air detection alarms
	Clamp venous line
	Stop the blood pump
	Place patient supine
	Call local emergency medical personnel
Air in dialysate	Venous chamber will trap small amounts of air
	Heed air detection alarms
	Clamp venous line
	Stop the blood pump
	Notify HHD unit
Water system problems	
Chloramine breakthroughs	Notify HHD unit
	Check activated carbon filters
	Check to see if municipal water treatment has changed
	(Continued)

Table 8-1 TECHNICAL COMPLICATIONS (*CONTINUED*)	
Problem	**Solution**
Low-pressure RO feed alarm	Install booster pump to the water line Stop other water-consuming equipment Use "flow-fed" RO
Abnormal water temperature	Install necessary cooling Use cooled heat exchanger
Maintaining water quality standards	Chloramine/Chlorine testing every treatment Product water and dialysate testing per unit policy Tap water AAMI water analysis prior to installation

AAMI, Association for the Advancement of Medical Instrumentation; HHD, home hemodialysis; RO, reverse osmosis.

a leak is detected, but this was shown to create additional burden and affected study participation.[10] A "panic button" or "alarm" is appropriate in certain situations of blood loss to contact local paramedics.

[For more information, see Chapter 3.]

Air Embolism

Air embolism is a rare but potentially fatal complication of HD. In a retrospective cohort study of 202 patients, air embolism resulted in less than one episode per 30,000 dialysis sessions.[9] Another study reported only a single case of air embolism among 190 patients over 11 years for an incidence of less than one episode per 100,000 HD sessions.[8]

There are three vulnerable areas for air entry:

1. Between the patient and blood pump due to negative pressure
2. Air in the dialysate
3. During connection to the dialysis circuit

Current HHD machines have sensors to detect air in the circuit, and to trigger an alarm and stop the blood pump in the presence of air. For air to enter the bloodstream, the patient would need to ignore or override these built-in safeguards. As a consequence of these advances in technology, air embolism in the contemporary era is usually a consequence of human error.

Air that enters the circulation can travel to the pulmonary artery, causing pulmonary edema, hypoxia, hypotension, and cardiac arrest. Air can also reach the central nervous system by entering the systemic circulation through a patent foramen ovale, or by ascending the internal jugular vein; this may cause altered mental status, neurologic deficits, seizures, and death. If an air embolism occurs, the blood pump should be stopped and the venous line clamped. The patient should be placed in a supine position immediately, and the care partner should contact local emergency medical personnel.

Water System Problems

Every component of a water system is essential for a successful HHD treatment. Water systems for HHD are more compact than those for CHD, but the quality of water created must meet the same standards. Monitoring of water and dialysate is necessary to avoid complications. Monitoring requirements vary by type of water purification system and clinic. Chlorine/chloramine contamination is the utmost concern—total chlorine levels are checked before each treatment (or after each batch of dialysate is made). Other chemical monitoring occurs less frequently for HHD than for CHD.[11]

Dialysate containing high levels of chloramine due to the smaller carbon filters in home water systems can lead to hemolysis or methemoglobinemia. Bacterial contamination occurs at a much lower frequency in HHD but water cultures must still be done per protocol. Water/dialysate containing high bacterial loads can lead to bacteremia or pyrogenic reactions (due to endotoxin). Other potential problems include extreme water temperature variations, which can affect the function of the water purification system. Cooling or cooled heat exchangers may be necessary in such situations. Low water pressure may pose a problem for reverse osmosis (RO) machines—installing a booster pump to the water line, stopping the use of other water-consuming equipment in the home, or considering a "flow-fed" RO system are potential solutions.[12] Any water system problem should prompt the patient to stop dialysis and call the dialysis center immediately.

[For more information, see Chapter 5.]

▍MEDICAL COMPLICATIONS

The summary of medical complications is provided in Table 8-2.

Hypotension

Intradialytic hypotension (IDH) is the most common complication during HD. It can be related to aggressive ultrafiltration (UF), inaccurate estimated dry weight (EDW), inadequate vasoconstriction, antihypertensive

Table 8-2   MEDICAL COMPLICATIONS

Problem	Solution
Hypotension	
Error weighing or calculating UF	Retrain with HHD unit
High UF rate	Utilize longer and more frequent HHD sessions Limit interdialytic sodium intake and weight gain
Incorrect EDW	Increase EDW
Cardiac factors	Utilize longer and more frequent HHD sessions Adjust dose and timing of antihypertensive medications with relation to HHD Avoid eating during dialysis Adjust dialysis prescription (i.e., cooling dialysate, increasing calcium in dialysate, etc.)
Access	
Access-related events	
Difficult cannulation	Nursing staff should review proper cannulation techniques
Inadequate clearance	Nursing staff should review proper cannulation techniques Check needle size Assess for proper needle placement Assess vascular access for thrombosis/stenosis
Bleeding around needles or prolonged postdialysis bleeding	Nursing staff should review proper cannulation techniques Assess vascular access for thrombosis/stenosis
Increased venous pressures	Nursing staff should review proper cannulation techniques Assess for proper needle placement Assess vascular access for thrombosis/stenosis *(Continued)*

Table 8-2 MEDICAL COMPLICATIONS (*CONTINUED*)	
Problem	**Solution**
Access-related infections	
Related to buttonhole technique	Use correct technique for eschar removal Consider prophylactic topical mupirocin Use correct aseptic techniques and "dry" times
Related to central venous catheter	Review correct hygiene technique Establish permanent access if appropriate
Loss of residual renal function	
Aggressive fluid removal	Set limits on UF rates
Electrolyte abnormalities	
Hypokalemia	Liberalize diet Replete potassium
Hypophosphatemia	Liberalize diet Add phosphorus to dialysate
Negative calcium balance	Adjustment of dialysate calcium
Nutrition	
Theoretical concern for loss of water soluble vitamins	Replace water-soluble vitamins
Sleep	
Insomnia	Address underlying medical conditions Provide sleep hygiene education Use behavioral and cognitive therapy Use medications where appropriate

EDW, estimated dry weight; HHD, home hemodialysis; UF, ultrafiltration.

medications, and other cardiac factors. Incorrect determination of weight and/or calculation of UF are standard errors in HHD often leading to IDH. IDH is defined as a nadir systolic blood pressure less than 90 mm Hg or an intradialytic decrease of more than 20 mm Hg with or without symptoms. Such a drop in blood pressure may have more severe consequences when it occurs in the home setting compared to the more controlled environment of CHD. IDH occurs when the UF rate exceeds the plasma capillary refill rate beyond the capacity of compensatory mechanisms such as increased vascular resistance and increased cardiac output. Excessive fluid removal is associated with detrimental outcomes such as myocardial stunning and increased mortality.[13] Greater intradialytic decline in systolic blood pressure has been associated with the development of regional wall motion abnormalities, and eventually a decline in left ventricular ejection fraction (LVEF). Three observational studies have demonstrated an association between greater UF rate and mortality; the mortality risk rises markedly above 10 to 13 mL/kg/h.[14]

In order to manage IDH appropriately, the HHD machine should allow rapid administration of intravenous fluids and reduction of the blood flow and UF rate. The patient should assume a supine position. More frequent HD (short daily hemodialysis [SDHD] or nocturnal hemodialysis [NHD]) allows for lower UF rates which reduces IDH, and should be considered for patients with significant IDH.

Other strategies to prevent IDH include:

- Adjusting dose and timing of antihypertensive medications in relation to dialysis
- Limiting interdialytic sodium intake and weight gain
- Avoiding eating during dialysis
- Adjusting dialysis prescription (using cooled dialysate, increasing dialysate calcium to 3.0 mEq/L, using sodium/UF profiling, using blood volume monitoring)
- Switching to peritoneal dialysis if refractory to other measures or have recurrent episodes.

[For more information, see Chapter 9.]

Access

Vascular access complications remain an important cause of morbidity and mortality in patients on HD. As many HHD patients dialyze more than thrice-weekly, they may have higher risk of vascular access events, infectious complications, and mechanical complications (i.e., stenosis, thrombosis, aneurysms, etc.).

[For more information, see Chapter 3.]

Access-Related Events

Vascular access-related events include difficult cannulation, inadequate clearance, bleeding around needle sites, increased bleeding after removal of needles, increased venous pressure during therapy, access loss, and access-related hospitalization. In randomized clinical trials, more vascular access complications were seen with more frequent HD. The Frequent Hemodialysis Network (FHN) Trial reported that the risk of a first-time vascular event for patients dialyzing with an arteriovenous fistula (AVF) was 1.9 times higher in the SDHD group compared to the CHD group (hazard ratio of 1.9, 1.11 to 3.25, $P = 0.017$).[15] The NHD cohort had a trend to shorter time to first vascular access event compared to the CHD group.[16] A similar trend of shorter time to vascular access-related events (both infectious and interventions) was observed in a retrospective cohort of 286 patients receiving extended HD more than 3.5 sessions per week ($P < 0.001$).[17] Sixty percent of the events were infection-related.

It is essential for nursing staff to review proper cannulation technique with patients regularly. Most patients stick needles in an antegrade fashion, as the needles should be visible. The needles should be at least 3 inches apart; all supplies should be kept within reach of the patient (including hemostasis supplies and a discarded needle container). Most centers recommend rotating needle insertion sites. Use of constant needle insertion sites (buttonhole technique) has been associated with higher infection risk, damage to the track from miscannulation, and longer training time. Vascular accesses should be monitored for infiltration and aneurysm/pseudoaneurysm development.

[For more information, see Chapter 3.]

Access-Related Infections

Infectious complications are a major source of morbidity and mortality in HD. In an intention to treat analysis of 3480 Medicare beneficiaries, the hazard ratio of access-related infection was 1.39 (1.28 to 1.50) for SDHD compared to CHD.[18] The excess risk may be related to increased frequency of dialysis treatments, that is, increased number of cannulations where bacteria may be introduced into the access. Central venous catheters have been associated with the highest access-related infection rates while AVFs have the lowest rates. Among central venous catheters, femoral catheters are more prone to infection compared to those located in the internal jugular vein. Nasal and skin colonization with *Staphylococcus aureus* and bacterial colonization of HD catheters are risk factors for systemic infection. Management of catheter-related bloodstream infection involves antibiotic therapy and removal of catheter in the following cases: tunnel infection, exit site infection, resistance to treatment, persistent bacteremia, and fungemia.

Arteriovenous grafts (AVGs) pose a higher infection risk than AVFs, particularly for polytetrafluoroethylene (PTFE) grafts. Difficult cannulation, peri-graft hematoma formation, prolonged postdialysis bleeding, and breaks in sterile technique increase the likelihood of PTFE graft infection at needle puncture sites. Infection of an AVG is often recognized clinically. Signs and symptoms of local infection may include any of the following: pain, irritation, tenderness, redness, warmth, diffuse or localized swelling, serous or purulent discharge, and skin breakdown. Newer strategies to prevent arteriovenous access-related infection include the use of cryopreserved human femoral veins in place of PTFE. AVG infection rarely resolves with antibiotics. Surgical revision or excision is almost always needed.

Some patients with an AVF may use the buttonhole technique for cannulation, which involves repeated sharp needle cannulations at the same site to develop an epithelialized track to facilitate easier self-cannulation for patients using blunt needles thereafter. In a retrospective observational study among 235 HHD patients, the incidence rate of septic dialysis-related events was three times higher in NHD patients using the buttonhole technique than in patients on CHD (incidence rate ratio of 3.0, 1.04 to 8.66, $P = 0.04$).[19] The utility of topical antibiotics among the participants was unknown. An accompanying systematic review revealed a bacteremia rate of 0.15 to 0.60 events per 1000 patient-days with buttonhole cannulation.[20] S. aureus bacteremia and fistula abscess were significantly higher with the buttonhole technique in a randomized controlled trial among CHD patients.[21] Furthermore, a retrospective observational prepost comparison study of topical mupirocin for preventing S. aureus bacteremia revealed a decrease in AVF infection rate from 0.23 to 0.03 events per 1000 AVF days with topical mupirocin (odds ratio of 6.4; 1.3 to 32.3, $P = 0.02$). This study led to recommendations by the Canadian Society of Nephrology to use topical mupirocin during buttonhole cannulation in a NHD patient.[22]

[For more information, see Chapter 3.]

Loss of Residual Renal Function

There is more significant loss of residual renal function when starting NHD compared to SDHD or CHD. Lower blood pressure associated with more aggressive fluid removal and lower use of renin-angiotensin system blockers is postulated to be one of the causes of this loss of residual renal function.[23]

Electrolyte Abnormalities

An optimal dialysate composition would adequately remove solutes (including phosphorus), normalize predialysis electrolyte abnormalities, restore acid-base balance, and prevent intradialytic cardiovascular instability.[24]

HHD may be associated with fewer fluctuations in the patient's intradialytic plasma concentrations due to longer and/or more frequent HD sessions. Longer HD sessions result in near equalization of plasma sodium to dialysate sodium toward the end of dialysis. If dialysate sodium can be adjusted, it should not be much higher than plasma sodium. With NHD, there is a risk of hypokalemia due to low dialysate potassium (2 mEq/L is the highest potassium concentration for NxStage System One).

Extended HD sessions have favorable outcomes on lowering serum phosphorus levels and tumor calcinosis.[25] The FREEDOM trial showed a statistically significant reduction in serum phosphorus level in SDHD. Approximately 73% of participants in the NHD arm of the FHN Nocturnal Trial were not on a phosphorus binder by the end of the study, compared to 8% participants in the CHD arm.[16] Similar serum phosphorus reductions were obtained in a Canadian randomized controlled trial; in addition 60% reduction in intact parathyroid hormone (PTH) levels were noted among the NHD group compared to 20% in the CHD group ($P = 0.003$).[26] Phosphorus removal may be so significant in some patients that they require the addition of phosphorus to dialysate to prevent hypophosphatemia. In addition, patients on NHD may experience a negative calcium balance and may need adjustment of dialysate calcium (if possible) to control secondary hyperparathyroidism (HPT) of renal origin. Excessively high dialysate calcium in NHD can lead to low bone turnover and promote calcification.[27]

[For more information, see Chapters 7 and 10.]

Nutrition

NHD liberates dialysis patients from traditional dietary restrictions. There is no data to support the occurrence of nutritional complications with longer, more frequent HD sessions. Serum albumin, protein catabolic rate, and total body weight at 12 months did not differ between CHD and NHD groups in the FHN Nocturnal Trial.[28] Loss of water-soluble vitamins remains a theoretical concern, with possible consequences including pyridoxine deficiency and thiamine deficiency. Continuing to replace water-soluble vitamins remains the standard of care. Some healthcare providers double the dose of water-soluble vitamins in NHD patients, but there is no data to support this practice.

[For more information, see Chapter 7.]

Sleep

Insomnia is the most common sleep disorder among ESKD patients followed by obstructive sleep apnea (OSA) and restless leg syndrome

(RLS).[29,30] Insomnia is common during the early initiation of NHD. Treatment of insomnia includes addressing underlying medical conditions (e.g., anxiety, depression, etc.), education about sleep hygiene, behavioral and cognitive therapy, and melatonin as well as benzodiazepines. Despite early insomnia and concern that nocturnal treatments (with alarms, blood pressure measurements, and other events) could worsen sleep quality, overall sleep architecture improves with NHD. OSA has an overall prevalence of 21% to 47% among HD patients.[31] Sleep apnea is caused by upper airway congestion during recumbency, uremia leading to destabilization of central ventilator control, and concomitant comorbid conditions such as obesity and heart disease. NHD can improve the apnea hypopnea index (AHI) in a dose-dependent manner as well as increase the pharyngeal size of HD as occurring with improved UF and decrease in pharyngeal wall edema.[32] Also, uremic neuropathy and myopathy are common in the ESKD population—NHD could increase the strength and endurance of upper airway dilator muscles and correct neuromuscular dysfunction in the upper airway.

[For more information, see Chapters 7, 11, and 13.]

❚ PSYCHOSOCIAL COMPLICATIONS

The summary of psychosocial complications is shown in Table 8-3.

Psychosocial aspects related to HHD play an important role in the success of HHD. Proactive professional support, peer support, respite care, travel support, and financial support from the HHD healthcare team must be a priority for patient care. Patients undergoing HHD experience mental health concerns that are not typically experienced by patients undergoing other dialysis modalities. Patients who dialyze at home may feel isolated. Support groups or time spent with others who dialyze at home can help reduce feelings of isolation among HHD patients and care partners. An alternative is an advocate "buddy" system that encourages current HHD patients and care partners to provide support to others. Ensuring that patients and care partners have access to respite care and other resources is critical.[33]

The idea of performing a very technical procedure at home may be overwhelming to many patients who may find the concept of being cared for by trained staff at a dialysis unit more appealing. When educating patients (both those who are not yet on dialysis and those who are on HD) about dialysis modalities, it is vital to address any preconceived notions about HHD. Education needs to be delivered early and often. This education can be done in a "transitional care unit" (TCU).[34] Emphasizing

Table 8-3 PSYCHOSOCIAL COMPLICATIONS	
Problem	**Solution**
Feeling of isolation	Support groups or spending time with others
	Advocate for "buddy" system
Feeling overwhelmed	Understand the patient perspective
	Provide pre-ESKD care/education
	Enable perspective patients to connect with current patients
	Refer patients to a TCU
	Provide adequate preparation for HHD
Maladaptation	
Poor coping skills	Understand the patient perspective
	Screen and treat for preexisting mental health conditions (anxiety, depression, and/or substance abuse disorder)
Non-adherence	
Non-adherence to dialysis treatment, medication, and/ or diet	Understand the patient perspective
	Involve a social worker
	Screen for psychosocial parameters
	Give clear instructions
	Schedule periodic telephone contact or home visits
Care Partner	
Care partner fatigue/dropout	Provide education/Training
	Understand the patient/care partner relationship
	Check on care partner during monthly visits
	Adjust treatments to fit lifestyle
	Expect modality change
	Provide respite care or temporary switch to in-center HD
	Consider solo HHD
Employment issues	
Training time	Take leave under FMLA
Work demands	Communicate with employer
	Set realistic expectations
	Involve social worker to help with coping and constructing a plan for work/life balance
	Consider NHD

ESKD, end-stage kidney disease; FMLA, Family Medical Leave Act; HD, hemodialysis; HHD, home hemodialysis; NHD, nocturnal hemodialysis; TCU, transitional care unit.

adequate preparation for dialysis will obviate many problems and help reduce complications.

Maladaptation

Certain preexisting conditions such as anxiety or mood disorders may be exacerbated when starting HHD and can lead to maladaptation and poor coping with new situations. It is crucial to identify such problems and manage accordingly. Results from observational and randomized controlled trials evaluating the impact of HHD on QOL have been heterogeneous. Overall, there appeared to be an improvement of perceived physical health (physical component score—RAND 36) in the FHN Daily trial as well as in the FHN Nocturnal trial.[3] However, overall QOL was not improved. Psychosocial assessments when evaluating patients for HHD may be helpful as well.

[For more information, see Chapter 11.]

Non-adherence to Treatment

HHD is a treatment method that requires adherence to dialysis treatments, prescribed medications, and dietary and fluid restrictions. Non-adherence to dialysis treatment results in undesirable consequences such as bone demineralization, pulmonary edema, and metabolic disorders, and leads to the development of cardiovascular disorders and ultimately death. A successful strategy for improving patient adherence must start with a multidisciplinary approach. Involvement of a social worker is crucial. He/she can inquire about the patient's social support system. Additionally, patients should be screened for anxiety and depression and given clear instructions and adequate training tailored to their particular needs. Teaching strategies for patients should include visual and auditory education materials. The multidisciplinary team may need to monitor and ensure adherence through regular telephone calls or home visits.

Care Partner Fatigue/Dropout

For most HHD patients, a supportive care partner is critical part of their success on HHD. The care partner may assist the patient in the HD treatment itself, management of HD-related symptoms, transportation to the dialysis unit and other medical appointments, management of diet, and maintenance of personal hygiene. These responsibilities may have a negative impact on care partners. The long duration/frequency of HHD and its potential complications can lead to stress and anxiety. Perception of unpaid care partner burden, as assessed by Cousineau self-perceived burden scale, was higher among NHD patients compared to CHD and SDHD (9.4; CI, 0.55 to 18.3; $P = 0.04$).[35] Care partner fatigue/burnout is a state of physical, mental, and emotional exhaustion.

During HHD training, it is essential to inform, educate, and adequately train both the patient and the care partner. Effective communication and management of expectations is key—this may prevent care partner fatigue. It is important to simplify the equipment and training process as much as possible to minimize retraining of patients. The staff must have a good understanding of the relationship between the patient and the care partner. Continuous vigilance is required to identify problems as they arise so that they can be addressed promptly. The patient and care partner should be given the option to adjust the HHD prescription to best fit their needs (e.g., reducing the frequency of treatments if needed or allow varying of length of treatments). It is also essential for the patient and care partner to understand that modality change is to be expected, and such transfers should not be considered a failure of therapy.

The patient and care partner should be provided with opportunities for respite care. Respite care is temporary or part-time care provided by a health professional or a paid respite care provider in the place of the care partner. This respite model is the most preferred as the patient's setting and dialysis prescription will not change, although it may not be available for many patients. Other options include dialyzing in-center HD for a short time or hiring a respite care partner to provide transportation as well as assist with other medical care at home.

In August 2017, the FDA approved solo HHD, where a trained and qualified patient may dialyze without a care partner. This may reduce the burden for some care partners without compromising the safety of the patient. Before initiating solo HHD, it should be determined that a patient is an appropriate candidate. Measures to ensure safety, such as prompt management of hypotension or bleeding, should be vigorously reinforced, as significant injury or death may occur if a patient becomes incapacitated and is unable to call for assistance.

[For more information, see Chapters 7 and 11.]

Employment Issues

For ESKD patients who work, balancing HHD (particularly training) with work obligations may be challenging. During HHD training, patients should be able to take advantage of the Family and Medical Leave Act (FMLA) to take time off and keep their job. FMLA allows 12 weeks of unpaid time off within a 12-month period. In addition, there are several laws to protect against job discrimination (e.g., Americans with Disabilities Act, the Rehabilitation Act and the Civil Rights Act). Patients need to communicate with their employers and have realistic expectations about the impact of HHD on their life and work schedule. Social workers at dialysis units may be able to help patients find ways to balance dialysis and work. Switching to nocturnal HHD may be a solution for some patients.

▌ REFERENCES

1. Saran R, R Bruce, Abbott KC, et al. US Renal Data System 2018 Annual Data Report: epidemiology of kidney disease in the United States. *Am J Kidney Dis.* 2019;73(3 suppl 1):A7-A8.
2. Culleton BF, Walsh M, Klarenbach SW, et al. Effect of frequent nocturnal hemodialysis vs conventional hemodialysis on left ventricular mass and quality of life: a randomized controlled trial. *JAMA.* 2007;298(11):1291-1299.
3. Hall YN, Larive B, Painter P, et al. Effects of six versus three times per week hemodialysis on physical performance, health, and functioning: Frequent Hemodialysis Network (FHN) randomized trials. *Clin J Am Soc Nephrol.* 2012;7(5):782-794.
4. Hladunewich MA, Hou S, Odutayo A, et al. Intensive hemodialysis associates with improved pregnancy outcomes: a Canadian and United States cohort comparison. *J Am Soc Nephrol.* 2014;25(5):1103-1109.
5. Lockridge RS, Kjellstrand CM. Nightly home hemodialysis: outcome and factors associated with survival. *Hemodial Int.* 2011;15(2):211-218.
6. Marshall MR, van der Schrieck N, Lilley D, et al. Independent community house hemodialysis as a novel dialysis setting: an observational cohort study. *Am J Kidney Dis.* 2013;61(4):598-607.
7. Weinhandl ED, Liu J, Gilbertson DT, Arneson TJ, Collins AJ. Survival in daily home hemodialysis and matched thrice-weekly in-center hemodialysis patients. *J Am Soc Nephrol.* 2012;23(5):895-904.
8. Tennankore KK, d'Gama C, Faratro R, Fung S, Wong E, Chan CT. Adverse technical events in home hemodialysis. *Am J Kidney Dis.* 2015;65(1):116-121.
9. Wong B, Zimmerman D, Reintjes F, et al. Procedure-related serious adverse events among home hemodialysis patients: a quality assurance perspective. *Am J Kidney Dis.* 2014;63(2):251-258.
10. Kennedy C, McGrath-Chong M, Arustei D, et al. A prototype line clamp for venous access bleeding in hemodialysis: a prospective cohort study. *Hemodial Int.* 2019;23(2):151-157.
11. Agar JW, Perkins A, Heaf JG. Home hemodialysis: infrastructure, water, and machines in the home. *Hemodial Int.* 2015;19(suppl 1):S93-S111.
12. Hamilton TE, Centers for Medicare & Medicaid Services. Survey guidance for a new home hemodialysis water treatment device, the "NxStage PureFlow™ SL Water Purification System (PureFlow™)". Published August 24, 2007. Available at https://www.cms.gov/Medicare/Provider-Enrollment-and-

Certification/SurveyCertificationGenInfo/downloads/SCletter07-34.pdf. Accessed June 22, 2020.

13. Burton JO, Jefferies HJ, Selby NM, McIntyre CW. Hemodialysis-induced cardiac injury: determinants and associated outcomes. *Clin J Am Soc Nephrol.* 2009;4(5):914-920.

14. Movilli E, Gaggia P, Zubani R, et al. Association between high ultrafiltration rates and mortality in uraemic patients on regular haemodialysis. A 5-year prospective observational multicentre study. *Nephrol Dial Transplant.* 2007;22(12):3547-3552.

15. FHN Trial Group, Chertow GM, Levin NW, et al. In-center hemodialysis six times per week versus three times per week. *N Engl J Med.* 2010;363(24):2287-2300.

16. Rocco MV, Lockridge RS Jr, Beck GJ, et al. The effects of frequent nocturnal home hemodialysis: the Frequent Hemodialysis Network nocturnal trial. *Kidney Int.* 2011;80(10):1080-1091.

17. Jun M, Jardine MJ, Gray N, et al. Outcomes of extended-hours hemodialysis performed predominantly at home. *Am J Kidney Dis.* 2013;61(2):247-253.

18. Weinhandl ED, Nieman KM, Gilbertson DT, Collins AJ. Hospitalization in daily home hemodialysis and matched thrice-weekly in-center hemodialysis patients. *Am J Kidney Dis.* 2015;65(1):98-108.

19. Van Eps CL, Jones M, Ng T, et al. The impact of extended-hours home hemodialysis and buttonhole cannulation technique on hospitalization rates for septic events related to dialysis access. *Hemodial Int.* 2010;14(4):451-463.

20. Mustafa RA, Zimmerman D, Rioux JP, et al. Vascular access for intensive maintenance hemodialysis: a systematic review for a Canadian Society of Nephrology clinical practice guideline. *Am J Kidney Dis.* 2013;62(1):112-131.

21. MacRae JM, Ahmed SB, Atkar R, Hemmelgarn BR. A randomized trial comparing buttonhole with rope ladder needling in conventional hemodialysis patients. *Clin J Am Soc Nephrol.* 2012;7(10):1632-1638.

22. Nesrallah GE, Cuerden M, Wong JH, Pierratos A. *Staphylococcus aureus* bacteremia and buttonhole cannulation: long-term safety and efficacy of mupirocin prophylaxis. *Clin J Am Soc Nephrol.* 2010;5(6):1047-1053.

23. Daugirdas JT, Greene T, Rocco MV, et al. Effect of frequent hemodialysis on residual kidney function. *Kidney Int.* 2013;83(5):949-958.

24. Locatelli F, La Milia V, Violo L, Del Vecchio L, Di Filippo S. Optimizing haemodialysate composition. *Clin Kidney J.* 2015;8(5):580-589.

25. Kim SJ, Goldstein M, Szabo T, Pierratos A. Resolution of massive uremic tumoral calcinosis with daily nocturnal home hemodialysis. *Am J Kidney Dis.* 2003;41(3):E12.

26. Walsh M, Manns BJ, Klarenbach S, Tonelli M, Hemmelgarn B, Culleton B. The effects of nocturnal compared with conventional hemodialysis on mineral metabolism: a randomized-controlled trial. *Hemodial Int.* 2010;14(2):174-181.

27. Al-Hejaili F, Kortas C, Leitch R, et al. Nocturnal but not short hours quotidian hemodialysis requires an elevated dialysate calcium concentration. *J Am Soc Nephrol.* 2003;14(9):2322-2328.

28. Kaysen GA, Greene T, Larive B, et al. The effect of frequent hemodialysis on nutrition and body composition: Frequent Hemodialysis Network trial. *Kidney Int.* 2012;82(1):90-99.

29. Merlino G, Piani A, Dolso P, et al. Sleep disorders in patients with end-stage renal disease undergoing dialysis therapy. *Nephrol Dial Transplant*. 2006;21(1):184-190.

30. Jaber BL, Schiller B, Burkart JM, et al. Impact of short daily hemodialysis on restless legs symptoms and sleep disturbances. *Clin J Am Soc Nephrol*. 2011;6(5):1049-1056.

31. Pressman MR, Benz RL, Schleifer CR, Peterson DD. Sleep disordered breathing in ESRD: acute beneficial effects of treatment with nasal continuous positive airway pressure. *Kidney Int*. 1993;43(5):1134-1139.

32. Beecroft JM, Hoffstein V, Pierratos A, Chan CT, McFarlane P, Hanly PJ. Nocturnal haemodialysis increases pharyngeal size in patients with sleep apnoea and end-stage renal disease. *Nephrol Dial Transplant*. 2008;23(2):673-679.

33. Nearhos J, van Eps C, Connor J. Psychological factors associated with successful outcomes in home haemodialysis. *Nephrology (Carlton)*. 2013;18(7):505-509.

34. Bowman B, Zheng S, Yang A, et al. Improving incident ESRD care via a transitional care unit. *Am J Kidney Dis*. 2018;72(2):278-283.

35. Suri RS, Larive B, Hall Y, et al. Effects of frequent hemodialysis on perceived caregiver burden in the Frequent Hemodialysis Network trials. *Clin J Am Soc Nephrol*. 2014;9(5):936-942.

CARDIOVASCULAR OUTCOMES AND HOME HEMODIALYSIS 9

Nasim Wiegley and José A. Morfín

Cardiovascular disease (CVD) is prevalent in patients with chronic kidney disease (CKD), and has been reported to be more than twice as likely to develop in patients with CKD compared to the general Medicare population.[1] CVD prevalence increases with progression of CKD, and is the leading cause of death in individuals with advanced CKD, particularly among those requiring dialysis. Left ventricular hypertrophy (LVH) is a maladaptive response to volume/pressure overload that leads to cardiomyopathy. LVH is quite prevalent in end-stage kidney disease (ESKD), with reported rates as high as 90%, and thus is an important predictor of CVD morbidity and mortality.[2] Anemia, mineral bone metabolism, uremia/inflammation, and most importantly hypertension (HTN) have all been implicated in the development of LVH.[3] As a consequence, the overall rates of CVD-related hospitalizations and mortality remain high in ESKD, despite a slight reduction over the past decade, pointing toward the need for interventions that improve CVD outcomes in this vulnerable patient population.[1]

The majority of patients with ESKD in the United States undergo in-center thrice-weekly hemodialysis (HD). This regimen of HD, typically 3 to 4 hours per session, is suboptimal as it is associated with significant hemodynamic instability, which leads to unintended clinical consequences. Many patients are in a chronic fluid overload state, which is also associated with worse CVD outcomes. Achieving euvolemia is challenging due to intradialytic hypotension (IDH) which is observed in at least 25% of outpatient dialysis sessions.[4] IDH occurs as a result of aggressive ultrafiltration (UF) in a relatively short period of time and the mismatch which occurs between the rates of UF and plasma capillary refill. The downstream effects lead to tremendous stress on the heart and other vulnerable vascular beds (such as those in the brain, gastrointestinal tract, and kidney). Foley et al. showed approximately 23% higher risk of death on the first day after the long interdialytic interval, and higher cardiovascular hospitalization rates after this long period.[5] This high-risk interval has been termed by some as the "killer gap," given its association with higher rates of cardiovascular-related hospitalizations and mortality (Figure 9-1). Intensive HD or more frequent HD offers an alternative for prescribers with a gentler option in the form of either short daily or extended nocturnal treatments, which reduces the interdialytic weight gain and promotes more favorable rates of fluid removal. Given the logistics and limitations of performing more frequent HD in the dialysis clinic setting, home hemodialysis (HHD) has emerged as a viable option to achieve better clinical cardiovascular targets. Given this premise, multiple studies on more frequent HD have demonstrated improvement in cardiovascular outcomes in the ESKD population.[6–10]

In this chapter, we review the epidemiology and the pathophysiology of LVH, an independent predictor of CVD, in ESKD patients, followed by a review of the literature regarding the beneficial effects of intensive HD or more frequent HD on CVD outcomes.

▌EPIDEMIOLOGY OF CARDIOVASCULAR DISEASE

CVD is the leading cause of death in the ESKD population with a prevalence rate of 70% in HD patients and 57% in peritoneal dialysis (PD) patients.[1] Heart failure (HF), coronary artery disease (CAD), and peripheral vascular disease (PVD) are among the most common cardiovascular diagnoses in the ESKD population. In 2015, nearly 40% of patients with advanced CKD carried a diagnosis of HF.[1] The high prevalence of CVD in the ESKD population is not surprising, given that diabetes and HTN remain the two leading causes of ESKD. The presence of diabetes,

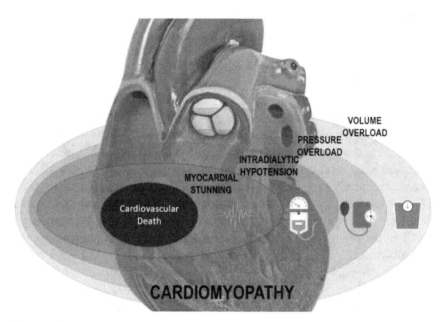

Figure 9-1 • Cardiovascular death mediated by volume overload and hemodialysis-induced stress.

HTN, and chronic anemia at the onset of ESKD contributes to the high morbidity and mortality in this population. Unadjusted cardiovascular-related deaths in the ESKD population have been reported to be 30 times higher than in the general US population. Compared to patients without CVD, ESKD patients with comorbid CVD have a higher 2-year risk of mortality, and CVD has been estimated to be the primary cause of death in approximately 41% of ESKD patients.[1] Foley et al. studied 32,065 participants in the End-Stage Renal Disease Clinical Performance Measures Project, a nationally representative sample of US patients receiving thrice-weekly HD. They observed an approximately 23% higher risk of all-cause mortality, and higher cardiovascular hospitalizations, on the first day after the long interdialytic interval.[5] Similar results were found in subsequent studies such as Dialysis Outcomes and Practice Patterns Study (DOPPS), and the United Kingdom Renal Registry.[11,12] Although these studies are observational in design, the consistent CVD morbidity and mortality associated with the long interdialytic interval in a CHD prescription has generated much concern about the consequences of LVH and the hemo-dynamic stress induced during HD.

LVH is a prognosticator of CVD, given its relationship to comorbid conditions that are associated with CVD.[2] Indeed, CVD and LVH are closely linked in the ESKD population.[6] LVH has been shown to be an independent risk factor for mortality in ESKD patients (relative risk of 2.9 for all-cause mortality and 2.7 for cardiac mortality).[2] LVH increases with progression of CKD and decline in kidney function; its prevalence is estimated to be 60% to 75% in the predialysis advanced CKD population, and greater than 90% in the ESKD population.[3] Furthermore, there is significant LVH progression in the dialysis patient. Foley et al. followed 596 incident ESKD patients without a history of CVD, and found approximately 62% developed increased left ventricular mass (LVM) index, and 49% had signs of LV failure after 18 months of HD.[7] In addition, in a prospective study of prevalent HD patients, increase in LVM index after 18 months of HD was significantly associated with increased risk of all-cause mortality and major adverse cardiovascular events.[13] Conversely, LVM index regression in patients with ESKD has been shown to have favorable outcomes on patient survival and adverse cardiovascular events.[14] Therefore, it is important to understand the pathophysiology and hemodynamic mechanisms at play to further develop management strategies of LVH and improve CVD outcomes in ESKD.

PATHOPHYSIOLOGY OF LEFT VENTRICULAR HYPERTROPHY

LVH is defined as an increase in LVM as a result of increased wall thickness. These structural changes are observed using echocardiography that further demonstrate impairment of ejection fraction and increased end-systolic and end-diastolic left ventricular volumes. Specifically, persistent volume and pressure overload lead to a compensatory myocardial hypertrophy, which compromises both systolic and diastolic function. This impaired ventricular filling leads to hypertensive systolic failure and cardiomyopathy that is highly resistant to the autonomic response[15] (Figure 9-2). The hemodynamic effects of both afterload and preload of the cardiac cycle are linked to the progression of LVH. Afterload-related factors are represented by an increase in systemic arterial resistance, elevated arterial blood pressure (HTN), and reduced large-vessel compliance related to aortic calcification (mineral bone metabolism).[16,17] Preload-related factors are linked to the role of intravascular volume expansion (volume and pressure loading), anemia, uremic inflammation, and the presence of arteriovenous fistulas which result in myocardial cell lengthening and eccentric or asymmetric left ventricle remodeling with activation of the intracardiac renin-angiotensin-aldosterone system.[17–21] The hemodynamic stress on the myocardium initiates several changes at the cellular level.

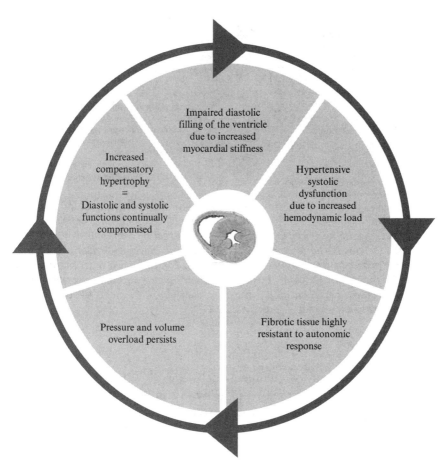

Figure 9-2 • The hemodynamic stress induced by volume and pressure overload on LVH. *(Modified from Advancingdialysis.org.)*

Activation of the renin-angiotensin-aldosterone system induces hyperaldosteronemia which promotes cardiac fibrosis through the generation of signals leading to profibrotic transforming growth factor production.[19] The myocardial cell lengthening is induced by the activation of cellular apoptotic signals and metabolic pathways that increase extracellular matrix production, leading up to fibrosis.[21,22] This fibrosis leads to progressive impairment in contractility with stiffening of the myocardial wall, systolic and diastolic dysfunction, dilated cardiomyopathy, and congestive HF.[23,24] It also leads to disturbances of cardiac electrophysiology because of ventricular electrical conduction impairment and predisposition to arrhythmias.[15] The LVH can also be further promoted by iron

Anemia:
- Erythropoietin deficiency
- Uremia suppresses bone marrow and can lead to inflammation
- Iron deficiency and ESA resistance
- Increase cardiac output preload

Inflammation:
- Diabetes
- Protein-energy malnutrition
- Development of atherosclerosis
- Poor response to ESA and iron handling
- Cardiac remodeling from uremia

Hypertension:
- Extra fluid and sodium retention in interdialytic period
- Over activity of sympathetic system
- Increase afterload and preload on cardiac cycle

Mineral Bone Metabolism:
- High phosphorus increases arterial stiffness from calcifications, increases afterload on cardiac cycle
- Hyperparathyroidism
- Metastatic and coronary calcifications
- FGF-23 role on cardiac remodeling

Figure 9-3 • Clinical contributors in ESKD to left ventricular hypertrophy and development of cardiomyopathy. *(Patrick J. Lynch; illustrator; C. Carl Jaffe; MD; cardiologist Yale University Center for Advanced Instructional Media Medical Illustrations by Patrick Lynch, generated for multimedia teaching projects by the Yale University School of Medicine, Center for Advanced Instructional Media, 1987 to 2000. Patrick J. Lynch, http://patricklynch. net, Creative Commons Attribution 2.5 License 2006; no usage restrictions except please preserve our creative credits: Patrick J. Lynch, medical illustrator; C. Carl Jaffe, MD, cardiologist. https://creativecommons.org/licenses/by/2.5/.)*

and/or erythropoietin or vitamin D deficiency.[25–27] These physiological changes to the left ventricle remodeling are influenced by key clinical mediators such as anemia, HTN, hypervolemia, disorders of mineral bone disease, and inflammation/uremia (Figure 9-3).

CLINICAL MEDIATORS IN LEFT VENTRICULAR HYPERTROPHY

Anemia is associated with compensatory changes such as reduction in afterload secondary to lower peripheral vascular resistance, and increase in preload from higher venous return, as well as increase in heart rate in response to elevated sympathetic activity. Chronic exposure to such changes results in LVH.[28,29] A meta-analysis by Parfrey et al. showed that correction of severe anemia (<10 g/dL) improved LVM index in ESKD patients on dialysis.[30] Another study by Chen et al. compared the effects or epoetin alfa versus darbepoetin alfa on LVH in subjects with CKD. Both agents were equally effective in lowering LVM.[26] The correction of severe anemia (hemoglobin < 10 g/dL) with erythropoiesis-stimulating agents (ESAs) has been shown to attenuate LVH progression; however, the achievement of hemoglobin levels > 12 g/dL does not help further reduce the LVM.[25] Lastly, the cardiovascular safety concerns of ESA in recent years has lowered the hemoglobin target in ESKD and thus predisposed patients to more significant anemia especially after an acute illness or hospitalization during which hemoglobin level frequently drops.

Mineral bone metabolism derangements in CKD have also been associated with the development of LVH. As already discussed, vascular calcification is an early hallmark of CKD-related hyperphosphatemia, which results in increased afterload. This process has been shown to eventually lead to LVH.[31–33] Furthermore, vitamin D deficiency has also been shown to play a role in pathogenesis of cardiac disease in patients with ESKD. Indeed, in observational studies, vitamin D therapy has been associated with lower frequency of cardiovascular events and improved survival.[27] In addition, several trials have shown that higher parathyroid hormone (PTH) levels (intact PTH levels > 500 pg/mL) are associated with failure of LVH regression.[34] Novel biomarkers such as FGF-23, a member of the fibroblast growth factor family, have been primarily implicated and involved in mineral bone disorder and secondary hyperparathyroidism.[35] In addition, the results of several clinical trials suggest a close relationship between FGF-23, cardiovascular mortality, and LVH.[36–38] However, we lack therapies that can directly modulate FGF-23. Therefore, strategies that target the calcium and phosphorus product remain the mainstay in the mineral bone metabolism domain. Given the complexity of LVH, aiming to mitigate the hemodynamic stressors on cardiac status and achieve appropriate volume status with dialysis appears to have the biggest promise and opportunity to improve CVD outcomes.

The prevalence of HTN is high in patients with CKD and increases with decline in kidney function. Results from the KEEP (Kidney Early Evaluation Program) and NHANES (National Health and Nutrition Examination Survey) studies showed greater than 90% prevalence of HTN in patients with advanced CKD stages G4 or G5 (estimated GFR <30 mL/min/1.73 m^2).[39] One of the main contributing factors to the pathogenesis of HTN is hypervolemia or volume overload, which is particularly problematic in ESKD patients with limited residual renal function on conventional thrice-weekly HD.[40–42] For instance, an analysis of participants in the CLIMB study (Crit-Line Intradialytic Monitoring Benefit) showed a direct relationship between interdialytic weight gain and rise in systolic blood pressure.[43] Furthermore, the DRIP study (Dry Weight Reduction in Hypertensive Hemodialysis Patients) showed that additional UF therapy reduced ambulatory systolic blood pressure compared to usual conservative management.[44]

HTN is associated with worse clinical outcomes including higher prevalence of LVH, as well as higher risk of mortality.[40,41,45] A meta-analysis

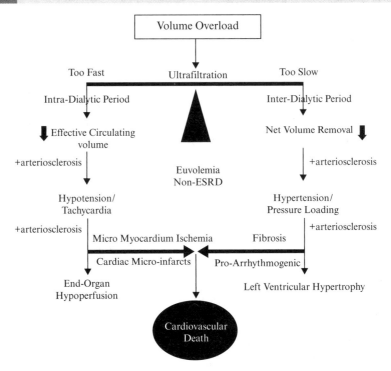

Figure 9-4 • Ultrafiltration volume interplay during hemodialysis and downstream effects on cardiovascular death. *(Created from Flythe JE, Kimmel SE, Brunelli SM. Rapid fluid removal during dialysis is associated with cardiovascular morbidity and mortality. Kidney Int. 2011;79: 250-257.)*

of eight randomized clinical trials showed that blood pressure lowering in HD patients with HTN was associated with lower risks of cardiovascular events (RR 0.71, 0.55 to 0.92; $P = 0.009$), all-cause mortality (RR 0.80, 0.66 to 0.96; $P = 0.014$), and cardiovascular mortality (RR 0.71, 0.50 to 0.99; $P = 0.044$) compared to control groups.[46] In a large international cohort study of nearly 40,000 incident ESKD patients, chronic fluid overload measured by bioimpedance has been associated with higher mortality risk compared to those individuals who are euvolemic.[47] Moreover, in the same study, the 1-year fluid overload exposure predicted a higher death risk across all systolic blood pressure categories, elucidating the importance of achieving a euvolemic state. Further in a population-based study, Kalantar-Zadeh et al. demonstrated that interdialytic weight gain greater than 2 kg was observed in 70% of HD patients and greater than 3 kg was observed in 40% of HD patients.[48] The common problem of volume overload poses a challenge in ESKD patients as it involves a two-pronged approach by combining reduction in interdialytic weight gain and carefully managing intradialytic UF rates (Figure 9-4).[4,50] Achieving a euvolemic state can be very challenging, given the limitations of conventional thrice-weekly dialysis, namely high interdialytic weight gains and UF rates which predispose to IDH.

[For more information, see Chapter 7.]

▋ INTRADIALYTIC HYPOTENSION

IDH has been defined by the National Kidney Foundation as a decrease in systolic blood pressure by 20 mm Hg or a decrease in mean arterial pressure of 10 mm Hg associated with symptoms.[41] Others have defined IDH on the basis of an absolute nadir in systolic blood pressure in the absence of symptoms.[49] The prevalence of IDH has been reported in 25% of HD treatments, although depending on its definition some studies have reported the occurrence to be as high as 70%.[51] This is often the result of aggressive UF in a short period of time and the mismatch which occurs between the rates of UF and plasma capillary refill. Moreover, in an observational study by Flythe et al., a nadir-based definition of IDH was found to be the best predictor of mortality compared to other definitions available.[4] IDH is associated with symptoms that at times limit patients' tolerance of dialysis and UF, such as cramping, headache, and light-headedness. However, the clinical significance of IDH is much more than these symptoms.

Among various causes of IDH, UF volume and rate are of great importance. Potentially more important than targeting an absolute dry weight volume, higher UF rates have been associated with more risk of IDH.[50] Flythe et al. found that UF rates greater than 13 mL/h/kg body weight when compared to <10 mL/h/kg body weight were associated with higher cardiovascular and all-cause mortality.[50] These observations have been seen in both prevalent and incident HD patients in the United States. Further, a secondary analysis of a large dialysis organization dataset, which used more defined categorized UF rates, suggested that even lower UF rates, that is, less than 8 mL/h/kg body weight, may be optimal.[52] Mortality risk was seen to increase incrementally, with 3% higher risk for each additional 1 mL/h/kg UF rate increase above 8 mL/h/kg body weight. Despite the lack of prospective clinical studies on the relationship between UF rates and cardiovascular mortality, deductive reasoning would support a more frequent or longer duration HD session in order to reduce interdialytic fluid gains, allowing for lower UF rates and less episodes of IDH.[53] This is especially relevant as IDH has been associated with end-organ injury such as myocardial stunning, cerebral ischemia, gut ischemia, and decline in residual renal function.[8,54–59] Further, IDH has also been independently associated with higher mortality risk.[53]

[For more information, see Chapter 8.]

▌HEMODIALYSIS-INDUCED MYOCARDIAL STUNNING

Myocardial stunning is caused by intradialytic hemodynamic instability that results from silent myocardial ischemia.[54] This relationship was first described in the 1980s when transient ST-segment abnormalities were shown on continuous electrocardiography monitoring during the interdialytic period.[60] This phenomenon is caused by repetitive episodes of myocardial ischemia that are cumulative and eventually lead to myocardial hibernation and fibrosis, resulting in fixed areas of regional wall motion abnormalities and irreversible cardiomyopathy.[8,56,61,62] As a result, the HD procedure, unlike PD, has been shown to increase risk of silent myocardial ischemia related to intradialytic hemodynamic instability. Over the past two decades, multiple studies have shown a decrease in myocardial blood flow during HD, leading to left ventricular regional wall motion abnormalities that can persist for hours to days after return of normal perfusion.[8] McIntyre et al., using positron emission tomography with its excellent specificity and sensitivity of tissue perfusion including myocardial blood flow on cardiac function, evaluated a subset of patients without CAD undergoing HD, and captured areas of induced segmental ventricular regional wall motion abnormalities, which resolved after dialysis.[61] In another study, serial echocardiography during HD showed that approximately 60% of ESKD patients developed regional wall motion abnormalities during the treatment.[63] These findings are consistent with stress-induced ischemia and associated with intradialytic relative hypotension.

▌THE CLINICAL BENEFITS OF MORE ▌FREQUENT HEMODIALYSIS

More frequent HD or intensive HD, in the form of either a longer duration of each session or more frequent treatments, is a strategy for prevention of IDH as it has been shown in clinical studies to reduce the degree of hypervolemia and improve HTN control.[64] Ayus et al., in a single center prospective cohort study, compared 26 patients on short daily hemodialysis (SDHD) to 51 patients on conventional hemodialysis (CHD). At baseline, there was no statistically significant LVM index difference between the two arms. After 12-month follow-up, LVM index decreased by 30% in the SDHD arm, without any significant change in patients undergoing CHD. In the same study, the mean systolic blood pressure declined significantly with SDHD at 6 months; however, no significant difference in systolic blood pressure was noted at 12 months.[9] In a feasibility study for the NxStage System One, participants on in-center thrice-weekly HD were switched to in-center HD 6 days a week for 6 weeks, and then transitioned to home HD 6 days a week for 6 weeks. Mean systolic blood pressure was 17.6 mm Hg lower during the in-center frequent HD phase and 23.9 mm Hg lower during the home phase compared to those in the weeks prior to study initiation.[65] Lastly, in the Frequent Hemodialysis Network (FHN) Daily Trial, more frequent HD with six times per week treatments, compared to conventional thrice-weekly HD, significantly reduced predialysis systolic blood pressure from 147 mm Hg at baseline to 139 mm Hg at month 2 and decreased further to 137 mm Hg at 10 to 12 months.[66] In addition, the number of antihypertensive medications per patient decreased from 2.2 to 1.4 with intensive HD and from 2.3 to 2.0 with conventional HD. In the FREEDOM (Following Rehabilitation, Economics, and Every day-Dialysis Outcome Measurements), a prospective study of SDHD, the percentage of patients prescribed no antihypertensive agents increased from 21% to 47%.[67] This decline in the number of antihypertensive medications and better blood pressure control with more frequent HD has been consistently an effective strategy to deal with volume and blood pressure management in ESKD.

Improved blood pressure and volume control in ESKD has translated to improvement in LVH in multiple clinical trials demonstrating favorable outcomes of more frequent HD compared to conventional thrice-weekly HD. As previously mentioned, in a non-randomized controlled trial comparing SDHD (six times per week for 3 hours each treatment) compared to CHD (three times per week for 4 hours each treatment), SDHD was associated with better optimization of fluid and phosphorus levels, as well as a 30% reduction in LVM index compared to CHD.[9] In another study, home CHD (three times per week for 4 hours each treatment) was compared with intensive home nocturnal hemodialysis (NHD) (nightly HD for 8 to 10 hours each treatment). This study also showed regression in LVM index, left ventricular end-diastolic diameter, posterior wall thickness, and septal wall thickness in the intensive NHD cohort compared to conventional thrice-weekly HD.[68]

The FHN Trial investigated effects of intensive HD by randomly assigning patients to six times per week and conventional thrice-weekly treatments for 12 months. The mean LVM decreased significantly by approximately 14 g in the intensive HD group compared to CHD that translated to a 12% reduction.[10] In a post hoc analysis of the FHN trial, a more pronounced effect of frequent HD on LVM regression was noted in participants with LVH (>132 g) at the beginning of the trial.[69]

The FHN Nocturnal Trial was a smaller study with limited sample size and randomly assigned patients to either six nocturnal sessions per week or conventional treatment. Although this trial also showed a reduction in LVM from 141 g to 132 g in intensive NHD group, in participants with echocardiographic data at baseline and at 12 months, the results were not statistically significant.[70] In contrast, the Alberta Trial, which also investigated LVM regression between patients randomized to frequent long HD at home (>6 hours, five to six nights per week) or conventional thrice-weekly HD, showed a statistically significant LVM reduction in favor of intensive HD.[71] This study also showed a reduction in systolic blood pressure, antihypertensive use, and serum phosphate levels in intensive HD participants.

In addition to LVM regression, intensive HD has also been associated with lower rates of IDH, and in turn lower risk of regional wall motion abnormalities and left ventricular dysfunction (Table 9-1).[8,10,70,71] This was not the case in the FHN Daily Trial, however. Despite significant reduction in the rate of IDH per dialysis session due to higher number of sessions per week, the overall rates of IDH were higher in the frequent short HD group (six times per week HD) compared to conventional therapy.[66]

[For more information, see Chapter 7.]

❚ MORE FREQUENT HEMODIALYSIS AND MORTALITY

The FHN Daily Trial showed a statistically significant lower risk of the composite outcomes of death or increase in LVM with frequent HD compared to CHD after a median follow-up of 3.6 years.[10] Investigators subsequently followed participants for an extended period after study completion, and found a significantly lower mortality rate in the frequent HD group compared to the CHD group (intent-to-treat analysis hazard ratio 0.54, 0.31 to 0.93; $P = 0.024$).[72] In contrast, the Nocturnal Trial participants experienced increased risk of mortality after a median follow-up of 3.7 years (intent-to-treat analysis hazard ratio 3.9, 1.3 to 11.8; $P = 0.010$).[70] It should be noted that the FHN Nocturnal Trial had a high degree of crossover between groups, and it had low statistical power for mortality comparison due to small sample size; therefore, interpretation of the results is limited.

Weinhandl et al. compared daily short HHD with conventional in-center HD in an analysis of the US Renal Data System (USRDS)

Table 9-1 SUMMARY OF CLINICAL STUDIES ON THE CARDIOVASCULAR-RELATED BENEFITS OF MORE FREQUENT/INTENSIVE HEMODIALYSIS (HNHD, HHD)

	HNHD	HHD	IHD
Hypertension/Blood pressure control Systolic BP	5%▼	7%▼	Referent
Left ventricular mass index	8%▼	12%▼	Referent
Occurrence of myocardial stunning	50%▼	25%▼	Referent
Regional wall motion abnormalities	38%▼	31%▼	Referent

HNHD, home nocturnal hemodialysis (6 times per week); HHD, home hemodialysis (6 times per week); IHD, in-center hemodialysis (3 times per week).

registry; results suggested modest improvement in survival in favor of daily HHD.[73] In another observational study using a separate analysis of the USRDS registry, Weinhandl et al. compared the risk of mortality with daily HHD and PD. The results of this study suggested that relative to PD, daily HHD was associated with lower risk of mortality and hospitalization in chronic ESKD patients. In contrast, patients who started HHD within first 6 months of diagnosis of ESKD had similar risk of all-cause and cardiovascular mortality and hospitalization compared to participants who started PD.[74]

There have been multiple smaller studies investigating mortality risk of frequent short and long HD with either in-center CHD or home thrice-weekly HD. The results of these studies are conflicting and controversial, likely secondary to low power and methodological limitations of these studies.[75] A randomized control trial powered for mortality is likely not feasible, given the large number of patients that would need to be enrolled and the high morbidity and mortality of the ESKD population, at nearly 20% per year. Therefore, observational studies and short-term clinical studies using intermediate outcomes, such as LVH, as discussed above will inform future prospective clinical studies.

▌REFERENCES

1. 2017 USRDS annual data report: executive summary. *Am J Kidney Dis.* 2018;71(3):S1-S8.
2. Silberberg JS, Barre PE, Prichard SS, Sniderman AD. Impact of left ventricular hypertrophy on survival in end-stage renal disease. *Kidney Int.* 1989;36(2):286-290.

3. Di Lullo L, Gorini A, Russo D, Santoboni A, Ronco C. Left ventricular hypertrophy in chronic kidney disease patients: from pathophysiology to treatment. *Cardiorenal Med*. 2015;5(4):254-266.

4. Flythe JE, Xue H, Lynch KE, Curhan GC, Brunelli SM. Association of mortality risk with various definitions of intradialytic hypotension. *J Am Soc Nephrol*. 2015;26(3):724-734.

5. Foley RN, Gilbertson DT, Murray T, Collins AJ. Long interdialytic interval and mortality among patients receiving hemodialysis. *N Engl J Med*. 2011;365(12):1099-1107.

6. McCullough PA, Chan CT, Weinhandl ED, Burkart JM, Bakris GL. Intensive hemodialysis, left ventricular hypertrophy, and cardiovascular disease. *Am J Kidney Dis*. 2016;68(5s1):S5-S14.

7. Foley RN, Curtis BM, Randell EW, Parfrey PS. Left ventricular hypertrophy in new hemodialysis patients without symptomatic cardiac disease. *Clin J Am Soc Nephrol*. 2010;5(5):805-813.

8. Jefferies HJ, Virk B, Schiller B, Moran J, McIntyre CW. Frequent hemodialysis schedules are associated with reduced levels of dialysis-induced cardiac injury (myocardial stunning). *Clin J Am Soc Nephrol*. 2011;6(6):1326-1332.

9. Ayus JC, Mizani MR, Achinger SG, Thadhani R, Go AS, Lee S. Effects of short daily versus conventional hemodialysis on left ventricular hypertrophy and inflammatory markers: a prospective, controlled study. *J Am Soc Nephrol*. 2005;16(9):2778-2788.

10. Chertow GM, Levin NW, Beck GJ, et al. In-center hemodialysis six times per week versus three times per week. *N Engl J Med*. 2010;363(24):2287-2300.

11. Zhang H, Schaubel DE, Kalbfleisch JD, et al. Dialysis outcomes and analysis of practice patterns suggests the dialysis schedule affects day-of-week mortality. *Kidney Int*. 2012;81(11):1108-1115.

12. Fotheringham J, Fogarty DG, El Nahas M, Campbell MJ, Farrington K. The mortality and hospitalization rates associated with the long interdialytic gap in thrice-weekly hemodialysis patients. *Kidney Int*. 2015;88(3):569-575.

13. Zoccali C, Benedetto FA, Mallamaci F, et al. Left ventricular mass monitoring in the follow-up of dialysis patients: prognostic value of left ventricular hypertrophy progression. *Kidney Int*. 2004;65(4):1492-1498.

14. London GM, Pannier B, Guerin AP, et al. Alterations of left ventricular hypertrophy in and survival of patients receiving hemodialysis: follow-up of an interventional study. *J Am Soc Nephrol*. 2001;12(12):2759-2767.

15. Ritz E. Left ventricular hypertrophy in renal disease: beyond preload and afterload. *Kidney Int*. 2009;75(8):771-773.

16. Mominadam S, Ozkahya M, Kayikcioglu M, et al. Interdialytic blood pressure obtained by ambulatory blood pressure measurement and left ventricular structure in hypertensive hemodialysis patients. *Hemodial Int*. 2008;12(3):322-327.

17. Martin LC, Franco RJ, Gavras I, et al. Association between hypervolemia and ventricular hypertrophy in hemodialysis patients. *Am J Hypertens*. 2004;17 (12 Pt 1):1163-1169.

18. Gross ML, Ritz E. Hypertrophy and fibrosis in the cardiomyopathy of uremia—beyond coronary heart disease. *Semin Dial.* 2008;21(4):308-318.

19. Steigerwalt S, Zafar A, Mesiha N, Gardin J, Provenzano R. Role of aldosterone in left ventricular hypertrophy among African-American patients with end-stage renal disease on hemodialysis. *Am J Nephrol.* 2007;27(2):159-163.

20. Xu X, Hu X, Lu Z, et al. Xanthine oxidase inhibition with febuxostat attenuates systolic overload-induced left ventricular hypertrophy and dysfunction in mice. *J Card Fail.* 2008;14(9):746-753.

21. MacRae JM, Levin A, Belenkie I. The cardiovascular effects of arteriovenous fistulas in chronic kidney disease: a cause for concern? *Semin Dial.* 2006;19(5):349-352.

22. Nishida K, Kyoi S, Yamaguchi O, Sadoshima J, Otsu K. The role of autophagy in the heart. *Cell Death Differ.* 2009;16(1):31-38.

23. Zoccali C, Benedetto FA, Tripepi G, Mallamaci F. Cardiac consequences of hypertension in hemodialysis patients. *Semin Dial.* 2004;17(4):299-303.

24. Dorn GW 2nd. Apoptotic and non-apoptotic programmed cardiomyocyte death in ventricular remodelling. *Cardiovasc Res.* 2009;81(3):465-473.

25. Ayus JC, Go AS, Valderrabano F, et al. Effects of erythropoietin on left ventricular hypertrophy in adults with severe chronic renal failure and hemoglobin <10 g/dL. *Kidney Int.* 2005;68(2):788-795.

26. Chen HH, Tarng DC, Lee KF, Wu CY, Chen YC. Epoetin alfa and darbepoetin alfa: effects on ventricular hypertrophy in patients with chronic kidney disease. *J Nephrol.* 2008;21(4):543-549.

27. Achinger SG, Ayus JC. The role of vitamin D in left ventricular hypertrophy and cardiac function. *Kidney Int Suppl.* 2005(95):S37-S42.

28. Metivier F, Marchais SJ, Guerin AP, Pannier B, London GM. Pathophysiology of anaemia: focus on the heart and blood vessels. *Nephrol Dial Transplant.* 2000;15(suppl 3):14-18.

29. Mozos I. Mechanisms linking red blood cell disorders and cardiovascular diseases. *Biomed Res Int.* 2015;2015:682054.

30. Parfrey PS, Lauve M, Latremouille-Viau D, Lefebvre P. Erythropoietin therapy and left ventricular mass index in CKD and ESRD patients: a meta-analysis. *Clin J Am Soc Nephrol.* 2009;4(4):755-762.

31. Chmielewski M, Carrero JJ, Stenvinkel P, Lindholm B. Metabolic abnormalities in chronic kidney disease that contribute to cardiovascular disease, and nutritional initiatives that may diminish the risk. *Curr Opin Lipidol.* 2009;20(1):3-9.

32. Marchais SJ, Metivier F, Guerin AP, London GM. Association of hyperphosphataemia with haemodynamic disturbances in end-stage renal disease. *Nephrol Dial Transplant.* 1999;14(9):2178-2183.

33. Hwang HS, Cho JS, Hong YA, et al. Vascular calcification and left ventricular hypertrophy in hemodialysis patients: interrelationship and clinical impacts. *Int J Med Sci.* 2018;15(6):557-563.

34. Piovesan A, Molineri N, Casasso F, et al. Left ventricular hypertrophy in primary hyperparathyroidism. Effects of successful parathyroidectomy. *Clin Endocrinol (Oxf).* 1999;50(3):321-328.

35. Kovesdy CP, Quarles LD. Fibroblast growth factor-23: what we know, what we don't know, and what we need to know. *Nephrol Dial Transplant.* 2013;28(9):2 228-2236.

36. Gutierrez OM, Mannstadt M, Isakova T, et al. Fibroblast growth factor 23 and mortality among patients undergoing hemodialysis. *N Engl J Med.* 2008; 359(6):584-592.

37. Amaral AP, Oskouei B, Hu M-C, et al. Fibroblast growth factor 23 induces left ventricular hypertrophy. *J Am Coll Cardiol.* 2012;59(13 suppl):E1059.

38. Mirza MA, Larsson A, Melhus H, Lind L, Larsson TE. Serum intact FGF23 associate with left ventricular mass, hypertrophy and geometry in an elderly population. *Atherosclerosis.* 2009;207(2):546-551.

39. Rao MV, Qiu Y, Wang C, Bakris G. Hypertension and CKD: Kidney Early Evaluation Program (KEEP) and National Health and Nutrition Examination Survey (NHANES), 1999-2004. *Am J Kidney Dis.* 2008;51(4 suppl 2):S30-S37.

40. Bakris GL, Burkart JM, Weinhandl ED, McCullough PA, Kraus MA. Intensive hemodialysis, blood pressure, and antihypertensive medication use. *Am J Kidney Dis.* 2016;68(5s1):S15-S23.

41. K/DOQI clinical practice guidelines for cardiovascular disease in dialysis patients. *Am J Kidney Dis.* 2005;45(4 suppl 3):S1-S153.

42. Inrig JK, Patel UD, Gillespie BS, et al. Relationship between interdialytic weight gain and blood pressure among prevalent hemodialysis patients. *Am J Kidney Dis.* 2007;50(1):108-118, 118.e1-4.

43. Reddan DN, Szczech LA, Hasselblad V, et al. Intradialytic blood volume monitoring in ambulatory hemodialysis patients: a randomized trial. *J Am Soc Nephrol.* 2005;16(7):2162.

44. Agarwal R, Alborzi P, Satyan S, Light RP. Dry-weight reduction in hypertensive hemodialysis patients (DRIP): a randomized, controlled trial. *Hypertension.* 2009;53(3):500-507.

45. Ruilope LM, Schmieder RE. Left ventricular hypertrophy and clinical outcomes in hypertensive patients. *Am J Hypertens.* 2008;21(5):500-508.

46. Heerspink HJ, Ninomiya T, Zoungas S, et al. Effect of lowering blood pressure on cardiovascular events and mortality in patients on dialysis: a systematic review and meta-analysis of randomised controlled trials. *Lancet.* 2009;373(9668):1009-1015.

47. Zoccali C, Moissl U, Chazot C, et al. Chronic fluid overload and mortality in ESRD. *J Am Soc Nephrol.* 2017;28(8):2491-2497.

48. Kalantar-Zadeh K, Regidor DL, Kovesdy CP, et al. Fluid retention is associated with cardiovascular mortality in patients undergoing long-term hemodialysis. *Circulation.* 2009;119(5):671-679.

49. Raja R, Henriquez M, Kramer M, Rosenbaum JL. Intradialytic hypotension—role of osmolar changes and acetate influx. *Trans Am Soc Artif Intern Organs.* 1979;25:419-421.

50. Flythe JE, Kimmel SE, Brunelli SM. Rapid fluid removal during dialysis is associated with cardiovascular morbidity and mortality. *Kidney Int.* 2011;79(2):250-257.

51. Sands JJ, Usvyat LA, Sullivan T, et al. Intradialytic hypotension: frequency, sources of variation and correlation with clinical outcome. *Hemodial Int.* 2014;18(2):415-422.

52. Assimon MM, Wenger JB, Wang L, Flythe JE. Ultrafiltration rate and mortality in maintenance hemodialysis patients. *Am J Kidney Dis.* 2016;68(6):911-922.

53. Chou JA, Streja E, Nguyen DV, et al. Intradialytic hypotension, blood pressure changes and mortality risk in incident hemodialysis patients. *Nephrol Dial Transplant.* 2018;33(1):149-159.

54. McIntyre CW. Effects of hemodialysis on cardiac function. *Kidney Int.* 2009;76(4):371-375.

55. Findlay MD, Dawson J, Dickie DA, et al. Investigating the relationship between cerebral blood flow and cognitive function in hemodialysis patients. *J Am Soc Nephrol.* 2019;30(1):147-158.

56. McIntyre CW, Harrison LE, Eldehni MT, et al. Circulating endotoxemia: a novel factor in systemic inflammation and cardiovascular disease in chronic kidney disease. *Clin J Am Soc Nephrol.* 2011;6(1):133-141.

57. Iest CG, Vanholder RC, Ringoir SM. Loss of residual renal function in patients on regular haemodialysis. *Int J Artif Organs.* 1989;12(3):159-164.

58. Jansen MA, Hart AA, Korevaar JC, Dekker FW, Boeschoten EW, Krediet RT. Predictors of the rate of decline of residual renal function in incident dialysis patients. *Kidney Int.* 2002;62(3):1046-1053.

59. Lee Y, Okuda Y, Sy J, et al. Ultrafiltration rate effects declines in residual kidney function in hemodialysis patients. *Am J Nephrol.* 2019;50(6):481-488.

60. Zuber M, Steinmann E, Huser B, Ritz R, Thiel G, Brunner F. Incidence of arrhythmias and myocardial ischaemia during haemodialysis and haemofiltration. *Nephrol Dial Transplant.* 1989;4(7):632-634.

61. McIntyre CW, Burton JO, Selby NM, et al. Hemodialysis-induced cardiac dysfunction is associated with an acute reduction in global and segmental myocardial blood flow. *Clin J Am Soc Nephrol.* 2008;3(1):19-26.

62. Braunwald E, Rutherford JD. Reversible ischemic left ventricular dysfunction: evidence for the "hibernating myocardium". *J Am Coll Cardiol.* 1986;8(6):1467-1470.

63. Burton JO, Jefferies HJ, Selby NM, McIntyre CW. Hemodialysis-induced cardiac injury: determinants and associated outcomes. *Clin J Am Soc Nephrol.* 2009;4(5):914-920.

64. Saran R, Bragg-Gresham JL, Levin NW, et al. Longer treatment time and slower ultrafiltration in hemodialysis: associations with reduced mortality in the DOPPS. *Kidney Int.* 2006;69(7):1222-1228.

65. Kraus M, Burkart J, Hegeman R, Solomon R, Coplon N, Moran J. A comparison of center-based vs. home-based daily hemodialysis for patients with end-stage renal disease. *Hemodial Int.* 2007;11(4):468-477.

66. Kotanko P, Garg AX, Depner T, et al. Effects of frequent hemodialysis on blood pressure: results from the randomized Frequent Hemodialysis Network trials. *Hemodial Int.* 2015;19(3):386-401.

67. Jaber B, Collins A, Finkelstein F, et al. Daily hemodialysis (DHD) reduces the need for anti-hypertensive medications. *J Am Soc Nephrol.* 2009;20.

68. Chan CT, Floras JS, Miller JA, Richardson RM, Pierratos A. Regression of left ventricular hypertrophy after conversion to nocturnal hemodialysis. *Kidney Int.* 2002;61(6):2235-2239.

69. Chan CT, Greene T, Chertow GM, et al. Determinants of left ventricular mass in patients on hemodialysis: Frequent Hemodialysis Network (FHN) trials. *Circ Cardiovasc Imaging.* 2012;5(2):251-261.

70. Rocco MV, Lockridge RS Jr, Beck GJ, et al. The effects of frequent nocturnal home hemodialysis: the Frequent Hemodialysis Network Nocturnal Trial. *Kidney Int.* 2011;80(10):1080-1091.

71. Culleton BF, Walsh M, Klarenbach SW, et al. Effect of frequent nocturnal hemodialysis vs conventional hemodialysis on left ventricular mass and quality of life: a randomized controlled trial. *JAMA.* 2007;298(11):1291-1299.

72. Chertow GM, Levin NW, Beck GJ, et al. Long-term effects of frequent in-center hemodialysis. *J Am Soc Nephrol.* 2016;27(6):1830-1836.

73. Weinhandl ED, Liu J, Gilbertson DT, Arneson TJ, Collins AJ. Survival in daily home hemodialysis and matched thrice-weekly in-center hemodialysis patients. *J Am Soc Nephrol.* 2012;23(5):895-904.

74. Weinhandl ED, Gilbertson DT, Collins AJ. Mortality, hospitalization, and technique failure in daily home hemodialysis and matched peritoneal dialysis patients: a matched cohort study. *Am J Kidney Dis.* 2016;67(1):98-110.

75. Suri RS, Kliger AS. When is more frequent hemodialysis beneficial? *Semin Dial.* 2018;31(4):332-342.

MINERAL BONE DISEASE IN HOME HEMODIALYSIS 10

Page V. Salenger

▌ DEFINITION OF MINERAL BONE DISEASE

Mineral bone disease (MBD) is best described as a syndrome that encompasses altered bone morphology and vascular calcification, as well as abnormalities in serum markers of bone activity. The older term of "renal osteodystrophy" specifically refers to pathological variants noted on bone biopsy in patients with chronic kidney disease (CKD); however, bone biopsies are rarely performed in a clinical setting and are used now primarily for research purposes. Typically, the incidence of MBD rises as CKD progresses to end-stage kidney disease (ESKD); however, the disease may not be clinically apparent until the patient is approaching imminent need for dialysis.

It appears that the inciting event in the development of secondary hyperparathyroidism (HPT) is phosphate retention, usually due to a combination of kidney disease (resulting in nephron loss) and high dietary phosphorus ingestion. In an effort to maintain phosphorus homeostasis, proximal tubule reabsorption of phosphorus drops, leading to increased phosphaturia. Rising serum phosphorus levels result in the following actions:

1. Reduction in serum calcium
2. Decreased calcitriol production via suppression of 1-alpha-hydroxylase
3. Transformation of vascular smooth muscle cells to osteochondrogenic smooth muscle cells
4. Increased fibroblast growth factor-23 (FGF-23), which leads to lowered calcitriol levels (also via suppression of 1-alpha-hydroxylase) and a negative feedback effect on PTH production

Increases in FGF-23 (a peptide) and loss of both alpha-Klotho (a protein cofactor in FGF-23 binding) and calcitriol are relatively early events in CKD, and often correlate with early and abnormal changes in bone morphometry. However, the beneficial effect of FGF-23 in stimulating phosphaturia and decreasing intestinal phosphorus absorption is counterbalanced by its inhibitory effect on calcitriol with resultant hypocalcemia and HPT. The net effect of persistent hypocalcemia is a negative influence on bone morphometry, and has been associated with cardiovascular mortality in patients with kidney disease. Probably not coincidentally, rising FGF-23 levels have also been correlated with mortality in CKD patients; the exact mechanism by which this occurs is incompletely understood. Hypercalcemia, which may be iatrogenic, has likewise been shown to contribute to both vascular and extraskeletal calcification. Changes in serum calcium, phosphorus, and parathyroid hormone (PTH) have implications for both the density and sensitivity of vitamin D receptors (VDRs) and calcium-sensing receptors (CaSRs). This may be one of the pathways by which serum biomarkers of bone activity also influence cardiovascular mortality.[1]

MBD in CKD is generally divided into three major categories:

1. Osteitis fibrosa cystica, characterized by high bone turnover with increased PTH levels
2. Adynamic bone disease, with low bone turnover and low PTH levels; incidence appears to be increasing in ESKD, likely due to increasing use of vitamin D analogues and calcimimetics
3. Osteomalacia, characterized by low bone turnover and abnormal mineralization (less common with declining use of aluminum-based phosphate binders)

These three types of bone disease can coexist, and the presence of any raises the risk of bone fracture. Unfortunately, PTH and alkaline phosphatase levels are not always a reliable guide to the type of bone disease present, and bone biopsy remains the gold standard. Updated Kidney Disease: Improving Global Outcomes (KDIGO) recommendations suggest that serial measurements of serum calcium, phosphorus, and PTH, along with DEXA scan, may be useful in predicting fracture risk and guiding disease management. Despite robust experimental evidence of the role of phosphorus in secondary HPT, the optimal serum level of phosphorus to reduce all-cause mortality has not been elucidated. The recommendation to restrict dietary phosphorus must also take into account the potentially deleterious effects on serum albumin caused by protein malnutrition, particularly given the inverse relationship between serum albumin and mortality in ESKD. Interestingly, patients on home hemodialysis (HHD), despite presumably higher protein losses in the dialysate, tend to have normal serum albumin with little, if any, dietary phosphorus restriction. As will be subsequently discussed, more intensive and frequent hemodialysis (HD) appears to accommodate a diet higher in phosphorus content, as well as the phenomenon of postdialysis phosphorus rebound.

▌VASCULAR CALCIFICATION

Serial measurements of calcium, phosphorus, or PTH do not appear to correlate with coronary artery calcification. A reliable and less invasive predictor of coronary artery calcification is warranted, given the high incidence and mortality due to cardiovascular disease (CVD) in CKD and ESKD. An older literature review found that older age and longer dialysis vintage were the main determinants of vascular calcification.[2] No relationship has been consistently noted between calcium-phosphorus product and vascular calcification. Some studies support a relationship between arterial stiffness (measured by ultrasound) and vascular calcification, which may partially explain the observed high mortality rate due to cardiovascular events in ESKD. Elevated levels of the uremic toxins indoxyl sulfate and p-cresyl sulfate have been associated with CVD and accumulate in CKD. In animal studies, indoxyl sulfate promotes vascular smooth muscle cell production and increased expression of bone markers such as Runx2 and osteopontin, similar to proposed pathways in the pathogenesis of calciphylaxis. Exposure to both indoxyl sulfate and p-cresyl sulfate in rats leads to increased mortality; whether or not prolonged exposure to indoxyl sulfate and p-cresyl sulfate in humans contributes to mortality (on the basis of endothelial dysfunction) remains a matter of debate.[3] Also unknown is whether HHD would reduce exposure to these poorly dialyzable uremic toxins, thus decreasing endothelial dysfunction, vascular calcification, and calciphylaxis risk.

Vascular calcification associated with CKD-MBD appears to manifest as arterial stiffness and deposition of hydroxyapatite in the medial layer of the vessel. This arterial stiffness provides the substrate for the development of left ventricular hypertrophy (LVH) and hypertension (HTN). The key initial step toward vascular calcification appears to be the transformation of vascular smooth muscle cells to an osteochondrogenic phenotype, thus leading to increased production and secretion of pro-calcification factors. In patients with kidney disease, this is then coupled with reduced inhibitors of calcification, such as matrix G1 protein and fetuin A. As previously noted, this sequence of events is strikingly similar to the pathophysiologic pathways believed to cause the development of calciphylaxis. Of additional importance is the link between vascular calcification and the occurrence of abnormal bone turnover and mineralization seen in CKD patients. The combination of elevated serum phosphorus, hypocalcemia, and the uremic milieu, along with a deficiency of calcification inhibitors, all contribute to a vicious cycle of vascular calcification and increased fracture risk from disordered mineralization and turnover of the skeletal structure. Furthermore, the type of MBD present may influence the degree of soft tissue and vascular calcification, not only increasing risk for CVD, but also raising calciphylaxis risk. It appears that patients starting dialysis with preexisting vascular calcification will experience more rapid progression of arterial calcification than those without preexisting disease.[4,5] This raises several questions:

1. How do we reliably assess total body calcium in ESKD?
2. Should we be regularly following coronary artery calcification score in ESKD patients?
3. Does more intensive dialysis (such as HHD) ameliorate the progression of vascular calcification, and if so, how should it be measured?

Regarding this last point, Chan et al. demonstrated improvements in vascular smooth muscle cell biology (as measured by proliferation, caspase-3 activity, and Runx2 expression) when converting 15 patients from conventional hemodialysis (CHD) (i.e., three times per week) to nocturnal hemodialysis (NHD) (five to six nights per week for 6 to 8 hours per treatment). In addition to improvements in vascular smooth muscle cell biology, early-outgrowth endothelial progenitor cells from NHD patients were able to induce angiogenesis in an ischemic vascular model to a degree similar to non-ESKD subjects. In contrast, endothelial progenitor cells from CHD patients did not show the same ability to promote neovascularization in an in vivo model. In fact, in this study, microvascular perfusion was directly correlated with dialysis dose.[6,7] Improvements in serum phosphorus correlated directly with improved vascular smooth muscle cell production (Figure 10-1).[6]

Since vascular smooth muscle cell apoptosis can lead to medial vascular calcification (via matrix vesicles–containing hydroxyapatite), it would logically follow that vascular smooth muscle proliferation will result in decreased medial calcium deposition. Whether or not increased dialysis intensity would ultimately result in healthier vasculature, translating into decreased morbidity and mortality remains a subject of debate. It may prove difficult to tease out a single factor, given the number of potential variables causing CVD in ESKD, as well as the complex interplay between those variables.

▋ PHOSPHORUS HANDLING AND RENAL DISEASE

In typical Western diets, phosphorus intake is 800 to 1200 mg/day, with 60% to 86% absorption across the intestinal mucosa mediated by the sodium phosphorus transporter NaPi-2b.[8] A single 4-hour high-flux HD treatment will remove approximately 1 g of phosphorus. An 800-mg tablet

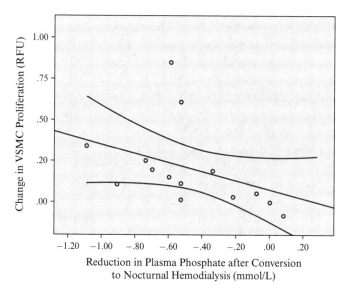

Figure 10-1 • Relationship between reduction in plasma phosphate and changes in vascular smooth muscle cell (VSMC) proliferation. (*Reproduced from Chan C, Lovren F, Pan Y, Verma S. Nocturnal hemodialysis is associated with improved vascular smooth muscle cell biology.* Nephrol Dial Transplant. *2009;24:3867-3871, by permission of Oxford University Press.*)

of sevelamer will bind ~26-mg phosphorus, and a 667-mg tablet of calcium acetate ~29 mg.[9] More recent research has demonstrated intracellular and paracellular pathways that govern expression of both intestinal and renal phosphorus transporters. In addition, the source of phosphorus—be it plants, animals, food additives, or medications—plays a role in both the extent and pathway of absorption.[10] However, the greatest rate of phosphorus removal on HD occurs in the first 60 to 120 minutes of the treatment, with some studies even demonstrating a rise in serum phosphorus before completion of the HD treatment. In healthy persons, phosphorus homeostasis is controlled by a combination of absorption of dietary phosphorus, bone mineralization, and varying degrees of phosphaturia. The proximal collecting tubule epithelium is the site of phosphorus reabsorption, and the percentage of reabsorbed phosphorus drops (along with increasing excretion) as serum phosphorus levels rise. Eventually, these compensatory mechanisms (which are accompanied by increased FGF-23 and PTH levels) will be overwhelmed by ever-increasing serum phosphorus.

A multipronged approach is usually taken toward controlling hyperphosphatemia in ESKD. This consists of three main cornerstones of therapy: dietary restriction of phosphorus, dialysis, and phosphate binders. Each of these has limitations and potential disadvantages. Strict dietary phosphorus restriction can lead to protein malnutrition; additionally, the "optimal" level of serum phosphorus that correlates with the lowest mortality in ESKD is not known. Use of phosphate binders is limited by their cost, relative efficacy, and side effects, all of which negatively affect adherence. Although some reports suggest non-calcium-containing phosphate binders result in less vascular calcification, this has not universally translated into better cardiovascular outcomes. Thrice-weekly HD, the mainstay of renal replacement therapy worldwide, is also limited in its ability to remove all dietary phosphorus over a weekly period. This is particularly true since length of treatment and frequency of treatment are the most essential elements of intradialytic phosphorus removal.[11]

In the Frequent Hemodialysis Network (FHN) trials, short daily dialysis reduced serum phosphorus by a mean of 0.46 mg/dL while nocturnal dialysis did so by a mean of 1.24 mg/dL.[12] As compared to CHD, short daily hemodialysis (SDHD) shows improved control of phosphorus; NHD as compared to CHD removes about twice as much phosphorus. Patients on four or more nocturnal treatments per week frequently do not require any phosphate binders, and are able to achieve this without any dietary phosphorus restrictions. Consequently, hypoalbuminemia is a rare event in NHD, and if it occurs, is often an early signal of an underlying pathological process. In fact, long nighttime treatments are so effective at phosphorus removal that some patients require phosphorus supplementation. With a regular, high-flow dialysis machine at home, sodium phosphate (i.e., Fleet enema) is added to the acid concentrate to yield a final dialysate phosphate concentration of ~1.0 mmol/L.[13]

[For more information, see Chapter 7.]

LEFT VENTRICULAR HYPERTROPHY AND CARDIOVASCULAR DISEASE

The differential effects of more frequent HD and in-center HD on serum calcium and phosphorus have potent implications for the development and regression of CVD, including sudden cardiac death (SCD) and LVH. Similarly, the influence of more frequent HD on FGF-23, its cofactor Klotho, and intradialytic calcium flux, and their relationship to mortality in ESKD, remain a subject of intense research. The exact mechanistic interrelationships of markers of MBD and their response to more frequent HD remain incompletely understood. Prospective studies have repeatedly shown the salutary effect of more frequent HD on the regression of both LVH and increased left ventricular mass (LVM) index.[14,15] As LVH, elevated FGF-23, and hyperphosphatemia are all associated with worsened survival in ESKD, the interaction of these variables with each other at the cellular level has taken center stage. More frequent HD has been noted to decrease FGF-23, phosphorus, and LVH, though results between studies are not wholly consistent. A study comparing 26 SDHD patients with 51 in-center HD patients reported a 30% decrease in LVM index in the former group; additionally, the SDHD patients experienced a 6% increase in serum calcium, 33% decrease in serum phosphorus, and a 42% decrease in median PTH levels. Despite the reduction in LVM index to more normal levels, blood pressure control was unaltered in the short daily group, suggesting other factors besides systemic pressure influence left ventricular remodeling. Some authors have explored whether changes in mineral metabolism are responsible for changes in LVM index. Hyperphosphatemia has been shown to predict improvements in LVM index, though this does not prove a causal relationship. Hyperphosphatemia is known to cause phenotypic transformation of vascular smooth muscle cells in the endothelium to osteochondrogenic smooth muscle cells, leading to vascular calcification, arterial stiffness, and reduced vascular compliance. Although this represents a tempting pathway to explain the link between MBD and CVD, the underlying pathophysiology is likely more complex and involves multiple pathways. NHD, while reducing serum phosphorus and LVH, has not convincingly demonstrated reduction in vascular calcification. FGF-23 is significantly associated with both mortality and LVH in ESKD.[16] As PTH induces increased cardiac fibroblast activity, FGF-23 is known to stimulate cardiac myocytes, likely through a separate FGF receptor (FGFR4) in the myocardium. This effect may be attenuated by administration of activated vitamin D, which paradoxically increases FGF-23 and alpha-Klotho expression.[17–19] What remains unanswered is whether more intensive HD will lead to decreased FGF-23 levels and reduction in mortality; the signaling mechanisms between FGF receptors and myocardial cells have been incompletely elucidated.

Multiple studies that have examined the changes in MBD parameters have documented little significant change overall in PTH measurements with more frequent HD. This is somewhat surprising, given the known beneficial effects of short daily, and especially NHD on hyperphosphatemia. Since patients dialyzing more frequently tend to have slightly higher serum calcium values, one would expect reductions in PTH; this is not consistently seen, and may be partially explained by non-adherence to activated vitamin D in the home setting. What is also unknown is whether longer dialysis treatments will result in lower FGF-23 levels, with subsequent "disinhibition" of PTH secretion.

The optimal phosphorus level in ESKD correlating with the lowest mortality is not known, though present Kidney Disease Outcomes Quality Initiative (KDOQI) guidelines provide a range, within which there is an association with lower mortality rates. Since phosphorus removal on dialysis is primarily a time-dependent phenomenon, NHD patients tend to have the highest weekly phosphorus removal; SDHD patients with treatment duration of at least 3 hours are the next best controlled group. NHD patients will sometimes require phosphorus replacement, while simultaneously maintaining normal serum albumin on an unrestricted diet. The key point is not only frequency, but also total weekly dialysis dose (i.e., intensity) to manage dietary phosphorus intake as well as postdialysis rebound of phosphorus. As previously noted, phosphorus removal tends to be highest in the first hour of dialysis; with significant amounts of phosphorus remaining in the osseous and intracellular compartments, phosphorus removal can drop off sharply during dialysis, particularly if the initial serum phosphorus was not greatly elevated. One study by Ayus' group in Texas showed that in-center HD removed 1572 mg/week of phosphorus, whereas SDHD removed 2452 mg, a 35% increase.[20] The Knowledge to Improve Home Dialysis Network in Europe (KIHDNEy) study in Europe, which utilized the NxStage system five to six times/week, but with only 2 to 3.4 hours/session, showed no overall change in serum phosphorus, though total weekly phosphorus removal was not measured.

There was also no change in phosphate binder use, perhaps due to the extremely short treatment times in a majority of the patients.[21]

In addition to determining the optimal prescription for phosphorus removal, more frequent HD and NHD both require an alternative approach to managing serum calcium. This is a potentially delicate balance: on the one hand, low dialysate calcium with subsequent relative and absolute hypocalcemia has been associated with prolongation of the Q-T interval and an observable increase in the risk of SCD; on the other hand, hypercalcemia and positive calcium balance are risk factors in ESKD for vascular calcification and calciphylaxis. In addition to the adverse effects of hypocalcemia (on bone as well as the conduction system of the heart) and hypercalcemia leading to calcification of vascular and soft tissue, the intradialytic calcium flux (i.e., the calcium gradient between blood and dialysate during dialysis) likely plays a role in calcium balance. This may be especially true in how fluctuations of serum calcium during dialysis affect the risk for cardiac dysrhythmias. Even slight changes in circulating levels of free calcium can influence the contractility of endothelial and myocardial cells. Acid-base status and levels of serum phosphorus also affect calcium levels; added to this is the difficulties in obtaining accurate measurements of serum calcium, whether by correcting for serum albumin, or measuring free calcium levels (Figure 10-2).[8,22–24]

[For more information, see Chapters 7 and 9.]

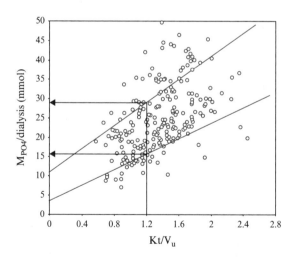

Figure 10-2 • Phosphorus removal during dialysis—relationship between dose of delivered dialysis (Kt/V_{urea}) and total mass of phosphate removed. (*Reproduced from Gutzwiller JP, Schneditz D, Huber AR, et al. Estimating phosphorus removal in haemodialysis: An additional tool to quantify dialysis dose.* Nephrol Dial Transplant. *2002;17:1032-1044, by permission of Oxford University Press.*)

∎ QUOTIDIAN (DAILY) HEMODIALYSIS

What is the effect of more frequent dialysis on the parameters of CKD-MBD? A number of trials over the past 20 years, originally designed to assess adequacy, blood pressure control, and mortality, have provided insight into optimal MBD management. This is seen particularly with regards to phosphate binder use and serum phosphorus levels. As previously noted, rising serum phosphorus levels signal an increase in FGF-23 secretion, resulting in decreased calcitriol production and lowered serum calcium. In turn, hypocalcemia stimulates PTH secretion, which can lead, if unchecked, to severe renal osteodystrophy. In addition to bone derangements, cost has become an issue: Medicare Part D expenditures in 2013 were approximately $700 million for phosphate binders, and $407 million for calcimimetics.[25]

The London Daily Hemodialysis Study examined the effects of quotidian HD in 11 patients. Although serum calcium, predialysis phosphorus, and postdialysis phosphorus changes were not statistically significant after 18 months, the calcium × phosphorus product did decrease; bone alkaline phosphatase and PTH rose slightly and phosphate binder use did not change.[26] In the short daily arm of the FHN study, 125 patients were dialyzed 1.5 to 2.75 hours six times per week. Higher serum phosphorus levels correlated with higher dietary phosphorus intake (with normalized protein catabolic rate, i.e., nPCR, utilized as a proxy measurement). On average, patients received 912 minutes of dialysis per week (vs. 639 minutes with thrice-weekly dialysis); mean serum phosphorus levels decreased by 0.46 mg/dL after 1 year, with the more profound drops noted in patients with a higher baseline serum phosphorus (Figures 10-3 and 10-4).[27]

In this group over 1 year, phosphate binder doses also decreased by 1.35 g/day; 81% of patients were dialyzed with a dialysate calcium concentration between 2.0 and 2.99 mEq/L. These patients also received increasing doses of activated vitamin D over the first year; PTH rose slightly, though not to a statistically significant degree.[27]

In contrast to the FHN study (which was done primarily utilizing large, high-flow machines), all 109 patients recruited to the aforementioned KIHDNEy cohort study dialyzed via the NxStage System One (which uses lower dialysate flow rates). The vast majority of patients dialyzed five or six times per week with a mean treatment time of 151 minutes. Patients dialyzing less than 15 hours per week had no significant changes in serum calcium or phosphorus levels; in patients dialyzing greater than or equal to 15 hours per week, there was a slight decrease in serum calcium and phosphorus, and a slight decrease in phosphate binder use, though not to a statistically significant level.[28] Although some of the shorter treatments (e.g., 90 minutes) were of the same

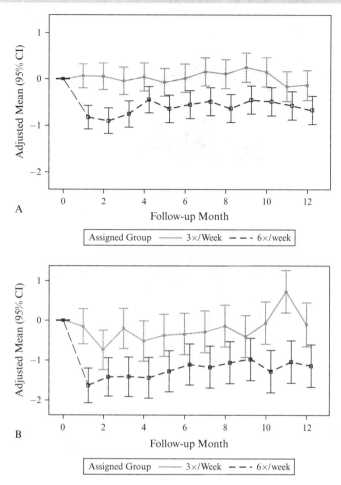

Figure 10-3 • FHN Trial: short daily and nocturnal arms: reduction in mean serum phosphorus levels with short daily (top) and nocturnal (bottom) hemodialysis. (*Reproduced with permission from Daugirdas, J, Chertow GM, Larive B, et al. Effects of frequent hemodialysis on measures of CKD mineral and bone disorder. J Am Soc Nephrol. 2012;23(4):727-738. Copyright © 2012 by the American Society of Nephrology; permission conveyed through Copyright Clearance Center, Inc.*)

duration as the FHN trial, perhaps the difference in dialysate volumes explains the differing results in phosphorus and binder use. Increased dialysis frequency would be expected to attenuate the effect of postdialysis phosphorus rebound; dialysis intensity (as measured by treatment time and/or volume of blood cleared) may be the more important variable. This is consistent with the observation that phosphorus removal is primarily a function of time, based on molecular size as well as its distribution among various body compartments. This is well illustrated in a Turkish study comparing 247 prevalent ESKD patients (selected in a non-randomized manner) who agreed to convert to in-center

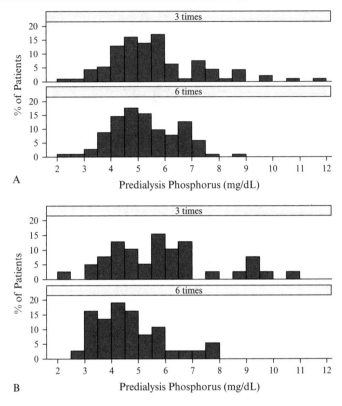

Figure 10-4 • FHN Trial: Conventional versus short daily (top) and nocturnal (bottom) hemodialysis arms: predialysis serum phosphorus levels. (*Reproduced with permission from Daugirdas, J, Chertow GM, Larive B, et al. Effects of frequent hemodialysis on measures of CKD mineral and bone disorder. J Am Soc Nephrol. 2012;23(4):727-738. Copyright © 2012 by the American Society of Nephrology; permission conveyed through Copyright Clearance Center, Inc.*)

nocturnal treatments thrice-weekly for 8 hours per treatment. They were matched to another group of 247 patients who continued to receive 12 hours of dialysis weekly (i.e., 4-hour treatments thrice-weekly), half the "dialysis dose" of the nocturnal group. In the NHD group after 3 months, there was already a significant separation as compared to the in-center HD group, with sharp reductions in serum phosphorus levels and phosphate binder use. Interestingly, in the same group, serum calcium rose slightly, but without measurable effect on PTH or activated vitamin D use.[29]

The ACTIVE Dialysis Study was a multicenter trial in four countries, randomizing 200 patients to either "standard" dialysis (12 to 16 hours per week) or "extended" dialysis (24 hours per week). Consistent with prior clinical studies, there were substantial decreases in average serum phosphorus per unit of dialysis time, as well as decreased phosphate binder use in the extended hours group.[30] Again noted was lack of measurable effect on PTH levels, despite a slightly increased serum calcium; perhaps a different mechanistic pathway to PTH regulation predominates in the setting of greatly reduced serum phosphorus. These results were achieved despite relatively lower blood and dialysate flow rates; the slight but significant increase in serum calcium in the extended hours group persisted even after adjustment for dialysate calcium concentration, serum phosphorus, and PTH levels. Additionally, in this group, there were several predictors of reduced postdialysis phosphorus: dialyzing more frequently than thrice-weekly, dialyzing extended hours in-center versus home (only 11% of the group), and a lower predialysis serum phosphorus. Normophosphatemia was maintained despite an unrestricted diet and reduced or absent phosphate binder use, with concomitant improvement in serum albumin. This is consistent with the observed association between serum phosphorus and mortality, as well as improved mortality rates in some studies of patients dialyzed for more hours per week. Because of its intracellular stores, phosphorus removal is more time-dependent than, for example, urea. Although a larger proportion of phosphorus is removed in the first 1 to 2 hours of dialysis, there is still ongoing phosphorus removal, albeit at a much lower rate, in extended hours treatment. In the ACTIVE study, the observed salutary effects of in-center (vs. home) extended hours dialysis was thought to reflect home patients' non-adherence to the dialysis prescription.

In contrast to the KIHDNEy cohort study, Ayus et al. examined phosphorus control in 26 ESKD patients receiving six 3-hour dialysis sessions per week, and compared them to 51 ESKD patients receiving three 4-hour sessions per week (i.e., 18 vs. 12 hours dialysis per week).[31] Patients receiving near daily dialysis saw reductions in average serum phosphorus from 5.02 to 4.20 mg/dL. The percent of patients in this group requiring phosphate binders dropped from 77% to 40%, while normalized protein catabolic rate actually increased. The differential increase in dialysis time of 6 hours resulted in a total weekly phosphorus removal 56% greater in the six times per week group. Hourly phosphorus levels, measured in 10 patients, did not differ in pattern between the two groups; all patients experienced the greatest removal in the first hour of dialysis. The generalizability of this study to the ESKD population as a whole is questionable; however, among the 77 patients enrolled in this study over 12 months, there were no deaths, suggesting their baseline health (and possibly residual renal function) were above average. Additionally, 92% of the patients were Hispanic, and at baseline, the patients who received near daily dialysis had lower serum calcium and much higher serum phosphorus than average. Since intradialytic phosphorus flux is greater with a higher predialysis serum phosphorus, were the observed decrements in phosphorus due to increased frequency of dialysis, or higher baseline phosphorus levels?

NOCTURNAL HEMODIALYSIS

NHD treatments differ from quotidian HD primarily in length; because of longer treatment times, frequency may be reduced, though "intensity" (as measured by Kt/V) is usually greater. A study by Kjellstrand et al. examining phosphorus flux in HD concluded that greater than or equal to 30 hours of dialysis per week was necessary to achieve normophosphatemia without binders.[32] Multiple studies illustrate the point that longer and more frequent dialysis (i.e., greater than three times per week) will impact a number of variables: dialysate calcium concentration, phosphate binder use, calcimimetic use, dose of activated vitamin D, dietary phosphorus ingestion, calcium supplementation, and even phosphorus supplementation. In turn, adjustments in these parameters can have far-reaching implications for clinical outcomes such as MBD, vascular and coronary artery calcification, and calciphylaxis. Since the typical American diet contains upwards of 2 g of phosphorus per day, and assuming maximal intestinal absorption (80%), the weekly phosphorus load could be as high as 11.6 g. Consider that the average in-center HD prescription removes approximately 3.7 g per week, while continuous ambulatory peritoneal dialysis (PD) removes even less, approximately 2.6 g per week for an average prescription. The other cornerstones of phosphorus removal also have limitations; dietary phosphorus restriction can cause low serum albumin, and phosphate binder use is limited by cost, side effects, pill burden, and non-adherence. Thus, it is not surprising that so many of our patients struggle with hyperphosphatemia. Hemodiafiltration and type of dialysis membrane do not appear to have significantly different effects on phosphorus removal. The more essential variables are dialyzer frequency and duration, membrane surface area, and predialysis serum phosphorus.

Mucsi et al. compared phosphorus removal in NHD versus CHD. Eight patients were dialyzed 12 hours per week (4 hours × three times per week) for 4 weeks, utilizing an F80 dialyzer with blood flow greater than 300 mL/min, dialysate flow 500 mL/min, and dialysate calcium concentration of 1.25 mmol/L. These patients were then transitioned to NHD six to seven nights per week for 8-hour duration. An F40 dialyzer with blood flow of 250 mL/min, dialysate flow of 100 mL/min, and dialysate calcium concentration of 1.25 mmol/L was used. Pre- and postdialysis values of serum calcium and phosphorus were similar between the two modalities; although phosphate clearance per treatment was similar as well, NHD was superior in total weekly phosphorus removal. In the nocturnal group over 3 months, serum phosphorus completely normalized and phosphate binder use was discontinued. Simultaneously, dietary phosphorus intake actually increased by 50% in the patients while on NHD.[33]

Al-Hejaili et al. followed calcium and phosphorus metabolism for 17 NHD patients for 18 to 24 months. As compared to short daily or CHD schedules, there were significant drops (on a dialysate calcium concentration of 1.25 mmol/L) in both serum calcium and phosphorus, occurring within a matter of weeks of initiation of NHD. Eventually all NHD patients discontinued phosphate binders. After 12 months, there were noticeable increases in both alkaline phosphatase and PTH, likely prompted by relative hypocalcemia. Dialysate calcium concentration was increased to 1.75 mmol/L with resultant decreases in both PTH and alkaline phosphatase toward normal. Calcium balance studies performed with a variety of treatment times and dialysate calcium concentrations concluded that patients dialyzing on a dialysate calcium concentration of 1.5 mmol/L or less will likely have net negative calcium balance, though this was somewhat dependent on dialysis duration. Those dialyzing with dialysate calcium concentration of 1.75 mmol/L would have positive (i.e., net gain) calcium balance. Not surprisingly, the four patients with a dialysate calcium concentration of 1.75 mmol/L also experienced profound decreases in PTH levels. Mass phosphorus removal per treatment was highest with NHD, and significantly more than with short daily or CHD. Removal of upwards of 40 mmol per nocturnal treatment (i.e., 1 g) enabled patients to increase their phosphorus intake without developing hyperphosphatemia. In fact, some of these patients developed hypophosphatemia and required either oral or intradialytic phosphorus supplementation. Conversely, long and frequent (five to six nights per week) dialysis with a dialysate calcium concentration of 1.25 mmol/L may lead to as much as 4 g calcium loss weekly, potentially resulting in negative calcium balance, hypocalcemia, and rising PTH levels.[34] In the above study, although PTH and alkaline phosphatase trended downwards after dialysate calcium concentration was increased, the decrease in bone biomarkers was not correlated with bone biopsy testing. The effect of NHD on PTH is quite variable, and largely dependent on fluctuations in serum calcium; other factors include vitamin D and calcimimetic use, dialysate bath concentration, and possibly vitamin D levels.[26]

Bugeja et al. retrospectively studied 39 ESKD patients who were "not optimally treated" by CHD; these patients were offered thrice-weekly, in-center NHD. They were dialyzed for 7 to 8 hours on slightly reduced blood and dialysate flows as compared to CHD. Over 12 months, mean serum phosphorus decreased significantly in the nocturnal patients;

PTH trended upward, but was not statistically significant. Elevations in alkaline phosphatase became significant after 12 months.

Ten nocturnal patients who were able to discontinue calcium-based phosphate binders subsequently became hypocalcemic; normocalcemia was restored when dialysate calcium concentration was increased to 1.5 mmol/L. Similar to NHD patients at home, these patients' rise in alkaline phosphatase was reversed by increasing the dialysate calcium concentration.[35]

Analysis of the nocturnal arm of the FHN study (where patients dialyzed six nights per week) showed that after 1 year, 73% of patients did not require phosphate binders.[27] In fact, in patients dialyzing more than 35 hours per week, 60% actually required phosphorus supplementation. In a conventional (high dialysate flow) machine, this has often been accomplished by adding 30 to 40 mL of Fleet enema to the acid component of the dialysate.[36] However, patients on low-flow (low-volume dialysate) devices do not have this option and will usually need oral supplementation. Similar to other trials of NHD, patients in the nocturnal FHN study required higher dialysate calcium concentration, usually between 1.5 and 1.75 mmol/L (corresponding to 3.0 to 3.5 mEq/dL); occasional patients required even greater than 3.5 mEq/dL. No significant trends were noted in PTH levels in the nocturnal patients.

From a biochemical perspective, calcium and phosphorus metabolism are important; clinically, how these variables influence MBD and coronary artery calcification are an even more essential consideration. Two studies from Australia shed light in regards to MBD management. Toussaint et al. retrospectively examined data on 11 NHD patients in Geelong, Australia. Patients dialyzed six nights per week for 8 to 9 hours, and had been on this schedule for at least 12 months before their data was analyzed. In order to follow bone density prospectively, DEXA scans were performed at baseline and annually thereafter. "Period 1" was CHD, "Period 2" was NHD with a low-flux dialyzer for a mean of 19 months, and "Period 3" was NHD using a high-flux dialyzer. Notable was the increase in dialysate calcium concentration to 1.75 mmol/L in the high-flux group, presumably due to increased calcium loss across the membrane. This change was made after development of osteopenia was noted by DEXA scans 12 to 24 months after starting NHD. Within a month of starting nocturnal therapy, all patients discontinued phosphate binders; when dialysate calcium concentration was increased from 1.5 to 1.75 mmol/L, calcitriol was also discontinued. In a small group of six patients with regular DEXA scans, improvement in osteopenia was noted after dialysate calcium concentration was increased. Postdialysis serum calcium levels, however, were relatively high, and remained so for up to 8 hours postdialysis.[37] It is unclear if this would result in increased ectopic soft tissue deposits or vascular or coronary artery calcification in NHD patients. This risk must be balanced against the marked improvement in hyperphosphatemia, in itself a risk factor for vascular calcification. One case report of a patient on NHD for 6 months demonstrated resolution of tumoral calcinosis and improved bone density.[38]

Toussaint's group in Australia retrospectively examined an additional 30 NHD patients from another center, for a total of 48 NHD patients. Once again, it was noted that in contrast to conventional or short daily dialysis, patients on NHD quickly became hypocalcemic and developed rising PTH levels with a dialysate calcium concentration of 1.25 mmol/L. The primary intention of this study was to determine if a dialysate calcium concentration of 1.75 mmol/L was preferable to 1.5 mmol/L in NHD.[39] Patients dialyzed 8 hours per night for five to six nights weekly, for a median duration of 32 months. Patients were divided into four groups according to dialysate calcium concentration and number of hours of dialysis per week (either less than or greater than 40 hours per week). Predialysis serum calcium and phosphorus levels were the same, regardless of time or dialysate calcium concentration. Postdialysis calcium levels were higher, and PTH levels lower, in patients dialyzing less than 40 hours per week on a higher calcium bath. At the same dialysate calcium concentration, these changes were not seen in patients dialyzing more than 40 hours per week, suggesting higher calcium loss across the membrane. From this, we can conclude that although postdialysis calcium rises with a dialysate calcium concentration of 1.75 mmol/L, at some point it returns to a lower predialysis level. The authors concluded that dialysis hours per week was the most essential determinant of postdialysis calcium level, with predialysis serum calcium also playing a role. Nevertheless, the differences were small enough that the authors could not definitively state a preference for one calcium bath concentration over another.

In addition to MBD, development of vascular calcification is another important clinical outcome. Hyperphosphatemia and hypercalcemia have been associated with cardiovascular and all-cause mortality, as has the incidence of calciphylaxis. Even alternate night NHD can control hyperphosphatemia without using phosphate binders in the majority of patients; subsequently, improvement in vascular and ectopic calcification and maintenance of bone mineral density are often seen.[40] To what degree NHD can reduce progression of vascular calcification and coronary artery calcification, and potentially impact cardiovascular mortality, is not known. Multiple studies utilizing electron beam or multislice computed tomography (CT) clearly show increased coronary artery calcification burden in ESKD patients; the predictive power of CT in ESKD to detect future cardiovascular events remains unclear. Yuen et al. followed prospectively 38 NHD patients, converted from either in-center HD, PD, or as incident patients. Coronary artery calcification was measured at baseline by CT, then 6 months and 1 year after starting NHD. Patients dialyzed between 30 and 48 hours per week; average age was 43 years and average dialysis vintage was 45 months. Unusually, only 18% of the study population was diabetic. NHD patients with no or minimal coronary artery calcification progressed to a nonsignificant degree; however, the studied population was young and had a low incidence of diabetes, which may limit extrapolation to an older and sicker ESKD population. In this study, serum calcium was stable, while serum phosphate and PTH decreased significantly. As we have seen previously, both phosphate binder use and antihypertensive medication use decreased with NHD, while vitamin D utilization was stable. Not surprisingly, patients with minimal coronary artery calcification had been on dialysis for fewer years, which may have biased the results of the study.[41] The nonsignificant rate of progression of coronary artery calcification in these NHD patients represents a lower calcium burden than progression seen in in-center HD and PD patients. A larger, randomized, controlled trial of longer duration would be needed to definitively determine if NHD is the preferred renal replacement therapy for patients at higher risk of coronary artery disease; for logistical reasons, this may never happen. Also unanswered is whether PD patients with serum phosphorus >5.5 mg/dL, who have a 2.4 increased risk for cardiac events, should be transitioned to HHD.[42] This observation could not distinguish between relatively low phosphorus removal across the peritoneal membrane and non-adherence of the patient to the prescribed PD regimen.

More information is similarly needed regarding the incidence of fracture in patients receiving intensive HD (whether short daily or nocturnal), and whether improved control of MBD would attenuate the risk of fracture. Additionally, if improved control of MBD results in slower progression of vascular calcification, would this translate into reduced incidence of peripheral arterial disease[43]?

Table 10-1 summarizes guidelines regarding management of MBD and the dialysis prescription in SDHD and NHD.

In conclusion, much remains to be learned regarding the potential benefits of HHD on MBD. More specifically, will longer, home-based, and more frequent HD lead to improved cardiovascular morbidity and mortality? Will improved phosphorus control contribute to both better cardiovascular outcomes and reduction in secondary HPT, as well as decreased incidence of fracture and calciphylaxis? If this can be shown, there may be long-term societal gains, with reduced Medicare expenditures on medications and emergency dialysis treatments; more importantly, our

Table 10-1	DIFFERENCES BETWEEN SHORT DAILY HHD AND NOCTURNAL HHD	
	Short Daily HHD	**Nocturnal HHD**
DCC	1.25–1.5 mmol/L; if using low flow machine (NxStage), use 1.5 mmol/L bath	1.5–1.75 mmol/L (3–3.5 mEq/L); with NxStage, use 3 mEq/L to prevent negative calcium balance. If using large machine, adjust accordingly. Avoid PTH over suppression.
Serum calcium	Unlikely to change significantly	More likely to develop hypocalcemia, especially if not taking calcium-based phosphate binders.
PTH/Alk phos	No significant effect	Either no significant effect, or more likely to increase in bone biomarkers secondary to iatrogenic hypocalcemia.
Phosphate binder use	Likely will need, especially if short treatment times, possibly at reduced dose	Likely can discontinue, even with unrestricted diet.
Serum phosphorus	Improved levels toward normophosphatemia	Marked decrease in levels; may even develop hypophosphatemia. If using NxStage, will need to supplement with increased dietary content ± oral supplements. If using conventional machine, can add 30–50 mL Fleet enema to acid component of bath.

Alk Phos, alkaline phosphatase; DCC, dialysate calcium concentration; HHD, home hemodialysis; PTH, parathyroid hormone.

ESKD population will be healthier, with potential gains in employability. Definitive answers to these questions have been hampered by the low recruitment of patients into HHD. However, given the current emphasis on increasing home dialysis, it is not unreasonable to hope that larger and longer trials of HHD can be undertaken to provide further guidance.

[For more information, see Chapter 9.]

▌REFERENCES

1. Qunibi W. Overview of chronic kidney disease-mineral and bone disorder. *UpToDate*. February 2019.

2. McCullough PA, Sandberg KR, Dumler F, et al. Determinants of coronary vascular calcification in patients with CKD and ESRD: a systematic review. *J Nephrol*. 2004;17:205-215.

3. Opdebeeck B, Maudsley S, Azmi A, et al. Indoxyl sulfate and p-cresyl sulfate promote vascular calcification and associate with glucose intolerance. *J Am Soc Nephrol*. 2019;30:751-766.

4. Moe S, Chen N. Mechanisms of vascular calcification in chronic kidney disease. *J Am Soc Nephrol*. 2008;19:213-216.

5. Shroff R, Long DA, Shanahan C. Mechanistic insights into vascular calcification in CKD. *J Am Soc Nephrol*. 2013;24:179-189.

6. Chan C, Lovren F, Pan Y, et al. Nocturnal hemodialysis is associated with improved vascular smooth muscle cell biology. *Nephrol Dial Transplant*. 2009;24:3867-3871.

7. Yuen D, Kuliszewski M, Liao C, et al. Nocturnal hemodialysis is associated with restoration of early-outgrowth endothelial progenitor-like cell function. *Clin J Am Soc Nephrol*. 2011;6:1345-1353.

8. Gutzwiller JP, Schneditz D, Huber AR, et al. Estimating phosphorus removal in haemodialysis: an additional tool to quantify dialysis dose. *Nephrol Dial Transplant*. 2002;17:1032-1044.

9. Sherman R, Ravella S, Kapoian T, et al. A dearth of data: the problem of phosphorus in prescription medications. *Kidney Int*. 2015;87:1097-1099.

10. Block G, Rosenbaum DP, Yan A, Chertow GM. Efficacy and safety of Tenapanor in patients with hyperphosphatemia receiving maintenance hemodialysis: a randomized phase 3 trial. *J Am Soc Nephrol*. 2019;30(4):641-652.

11. Kuhlmann MK. Management of hyperphosphatemia. *Hemodial Int*. 2006; 10(4):338-345.

12. Ketteler M, Wuthrich RP, Floege J. Management of hyperphosphatemia in chronic kidney disease—challenges and solutions. *Clin Kidney J*. 2013;6(2):128-136.

13. Perl J, Chan C. Home hemodialysis: daily hemodialysis and nocturnal hemodialysis: Core Curriculum 2009. *Am J Kidney Dis*. 2009;54(6):1171-1184.

14. Ayus JC, Mizani MR, Achinger SC, et al. Effects of short daily versus conventional hemodialysis on left ventricular hypertrophy and inflammatory markers: a prospective, controlled study. *J Am Soc Nephrol*. 2005;16:2778-2788.

15. Walsh M, Culleton B, Tonelli M, et al. A systematic review of the effect of nocturnal hemodialysis on blood pressure, left ventricular hypertrophy, anemia, mineral metabolism, and health-related quality of life. *Kidney Int*. 2005;67:1500-1508.

16. Gutierrez OM, Mannstadt M, Isakova T, et al. Fibroblast growth factor 23 and mortality among patients undergoing hemodialysis. *N Engl J Med*. 2008;359:584-592.

17. Grabner A, Amarel AP, Schramm K, et al. Activation of cardiac fibroblast growth factor receptor 4 causes left ventricular hypertrophy. *Cell Metab*. 2015;22(6):1020-1032.

18. McCullough PA, Chan C, Weinhandl ED, et al. Intensive hemodialysis, left ventricular hypertrophy, and cardiovascular disease. *Am J Kidney Dis.* 2016;68 (5 suppl 1):S5-S14.
19. Vervloet MG. Chronic kidney disease mineral and bone disorder: changing insights form changing parameters? *Nephrol Dial Transplant.* 2020;35(3):385-389.
20. Ayus JC, Achinger SG. Left ventricular hypertrophy: is hyperphosphatemia among dialysis patients a risk factor? *J Am Soc Nephrol.* 2006;17:S255-S261.
21. Cherukuri S, Bajo M, Colussi G, et al. Home hemodialysis treatment and outcomes: retrospective analysis of the Knowledge to Improve Home Dialysis Network in Europe (KIHDNEy) Cohort. *BMC Nephrol.* 2018;19(1):262.
22. Pun PH, Horton JR, Middleton JP. Dialysate calcium concentration and the risk of sudden cardiac arrest in hemodialysis patients. *Clin J Am Soc Nephrol.* 2013;8(5):797-803.
23. Makar M, Pun PH. Sudden cardiac death among hemodialysis patients. *Am J Kidney Dis.* 2017;69(5):684-695.
24. Kim ED, Parekh RS. Calcium and sudden death in ESRD. *Semin Dial.* 2015;28(6):624-635.
25. United States Renal Data System. 2015 USRDS Annual Data Report: Epidemiology of kidney disease in the United States. National Institutes of Health, National Institute of Diabetes and Digestive and Kidney Diseases, Bethesda, MD, 2015.
26. Lindsay RM, Alhejaili F, Nesrallah G, et al. Calcium and phosphate balance with quotidian hemodialysis. *Am J Kidney Dis.* 2003;42(1 suppl):24-29.
27. Daugirdas J, Chertow GM, Larive B, et al. Effects of frequent hemodialysis on measures of CKD mineral and bone disorder. *J Am Soc Nephrol.* 2012;23(4):727-738.
28. Slon M, Ficheux M, Fessi H, et al. Mineral and bone disease parameters on home hemodialysis with the NxStage System One. *Nephrol Dial Transplant.* 2017;32(3):iii 689.
29. OK E, Duman S, Asci G, et al. Comparison of 4- and 8-hour dialysis sessions in thrice-weekly in-centre haemodialysis. *Nephrol Dial Transplant.* 2011;26:1287-1296.
30. Zhan Z, Smyth B, Toussaint N, et al Effect of extended hours dialysis on markers of chronic kidney disease-mineral and bone disorder in the ACTIVE dialysis study. *BMC Nephrol.* 2019;20:258.
31. Ayus JC, Achinger SC, Mizani MR, et al. Phosphorus balance and mineral metabolism with 3-hour daily hemodialysis. *Kidney Int.* 2007;71:336-342.
32. Kjellstrand C, Ing TS, Kjellstrand PT, et al. Phosphorus dynamics during hemodialysis. *Hemodial Int.* 2011;15(2):226-233.
33. Mucsi I, Hercz G, Uldall R, et al. Control of serum phosphate without any phosphate binders in patients treated with nocturnal hemodialysis. *Kidney Int.* 1998;53:1399-1404.
34. Al-Hejaili F, Kortas C, Leitch R, et al. Nocturnal but not short hours quotidian hemodialysis requires an elevated dialysate calcium concentration. *J Am Soc Nephrol.* 2003;14:2322-2328.

35. Bugeja A, Dacouris N, Thomas A, et al. In-center nocturnal hemodialysis: another option in the management of chronic kidney disease. *Clin J Am Soc Nephrol*. 2009;4:778-783.

36. Lockridge R, Cornelis T, Van Eps C. Prescriptions for home hemodialysis. *Hemodial Int*. 2015;19:S112-S127.

37. Toussaint N, Boddington J, Simmonds R, et al. Calcium phosphate metabolism and bone mineral density with nocturnal hemodialysis. *Hemodial Int*. 2006;10:280-286.

38. Kim SJ, Goldstein M, Szabo T, et al. Resolution of soft tissue calcification and improvement of bone density on nocturnal hemodialysis: a case report. *Am J Kidney Dis*. 2003;41(3):E12.

39. Toussaint N, Polkinghorne KR, Kerr PG, et al. Comparison between different dialysate calcium concentrations in nocturnal hemodialysis. *Hemodial Int*. 2007;11:217-224.

40. VanEps CL, Jeffries JK, Anderson JA, et al. Mineral metabolism, bone histomorphometry and vascular calcification in alternate night nocturnal haemodialysis. *Nephrology (Carlton)*. 2007;12(3):224-233.

41. Yuen D, Pierratos A, Richardson RMA, et al. The natural history of coronary calcification progression in a cohort of nocturnal haemodialysis patients. *Nephrol Dial Transplant*. 2006;21(5):1407-1412.

42. Copland M, Komenda P, Weinhandl E, et al. Intensive hemodialysis, mineral and bone disorder, and phosphate binder use. *Am J Kidney Dis*. 2016;68 (5 suppl 1):S24-S32.

43. Nesrallah G, Mustafa RA, MacRae J, et al. Canadian Society of Nephrology guidelines for the management of patients with ESRD treated with intensive hemodialysis. *Am J Kidney Dis*. 2013;62(1):187-198.

QUALITY OF LIFE AND HOME HEMODIALYSIS 11

Emaad M. Abdel-Rahman

Quality of life (QOL) is a term that reflects the expectations of an individual or society for a good life. These expectations may differ based on the individual's values, goals and sociocultural context in which she or he lives. It is crucial for clinicians to understand their patients' values. High-quality clinician-patient decision-making is one of the cornerstones in chronic disease management, and when done well, patient-centered decision-making improves satisfaction, adherence, and ultimately QOL.[1] QOL involves several domains that subjectively covers the emotional, physical, material, and social well-being of an individual. It is now recognized that QOL correlates with survival of patients.

End-stage kidney disease (ESKD) is an irreversible chronic disease and is associated with significantly poor QOL, ranking among the worst of any chronic medical condition.[2] Poor QOL in patients with ESKD is associated with increased risk of mortality and hospitalization.[3] Multiple factors contribute to the low QOL of dialysis patients including medical, social, psychological, and financial factors.

Several management options are available for patients with ESKD, including dialysis, transplantation, or conservative management. Each of the dialysis modalities (peritoneal dialysis, in-center hemodialysis, home hemodialysis) and transplant offer particular benefits and challenges that lead to different levels of QOL. The change in QOL of patients on dialysis extends to their care partners with significant burden on their lives. The QOL of care partners differs depending on the renal replacement therapy (RRT) modality. Higher care partner burden score was observed in the care partners of in-center hemodialysis (HD) patients than those of peritoneal dialysis (PD) or kidney transplant patients.[4,5]

In this chapter, we will focus on the QOL of patients with ESKD on home hemodialysis (HHD), compare it with QOL of patients with ESKD managed by other RRT modalities and shed some light on the QOL of care partners of patients on HHD.

▌TOOLS TO ASSESS QUALITY OF LIFE

QOL outcomes can be measured using a variety of tools that are either disease specific or more general health or utility, such as the 36-item Short Form questionnaire (SF-36).

General

The standard approach to reporting QOL is through patient-reported experience (satisfaction scores) and outcome measures (health and functional status and well-being). The health-related quality of life (Hr-QOL) questionnaire includes several variables: survival and life expectancy; various symptom states; numerous physiologic states such as blood pressure or glucose level; physical function states such as mobility and ambulation, sensory functioning, sexual functioning; emotional and cognitive function status such as anxiety and depression or positive well-being; perceptions about present and future health; and satisfaction with healthcare.[6]

Kidney Disease

The disease-specific tool most commonly used in kidney disease is the Kidney Disease Quality of Life 36-Item Short Form Survey (KDQOL-36).[7,8] The KDQOL-36 augments the Short Form-12 generic core with 24 items used to score three kidney-specific scales: Burden of Kidney Disease, Symptoms/Problems of Kidney Disease, and Effects of Kidney Disease.

∎ HOME HEMODIALYSIS AND QUALITY OF LIFE

HHD is a form of HD that occurs in the home setting with an increased frequency compared to conventional thrice-weekly hemodialysis (CHD). HHD can be done as short daily hemodialysis (SDHD) or nocturnal hemodialysis (NHD). HHD is associated with multiple benefits to the patients[9–14]:

- Increased flexibility
- Schedule independence
- Decreased travel time
- Increased autonomy
- Fewer cardiovascular-related hospitalizations
- Decreased intradialytic weight gains
- Greater clearance of middle-sized molecules
- Improved mineral metabolism
- Reduction in left ventricular mass index
- Improved survival.

In fact, Pauly et al. showed that while survival of patients on NHD ($N = 177$) was inferior to patients receiving a kidney transplant from a living donor, it was comparable to that of deceased donor kidney transplant patients.[15] Despite these benefits, patients on HHD face numerous challenges and limitations including:

- More frequent use of their vascular access may contribute to loss of vascular access
- Increased likelihood of infection and increased hospitalizations for access-related infections
- Earlier loss of residual renal function
- More financial burden with higher water/electric bills
- Feelings of isolation, anxiety, and fear.

[For more information, see Chapter 7.]

Quality of Life of Patients on Home Hemodialysis

Several studies have assessed the QOL of patients on HHD. Mohr et al. reviewed data derived from studies carried out between 1997 and 1999 on patients with ESKD on HHD and CHD ($N = 197$). This review showed that daily dialysis was associated with improvement in several QOL parameters as compared to patients on CHD.[16]

Two subsequent studies in 2003 confirmed these results. Heidenheim et al. compared QOL between patients on SDHD ($N = 11$) and NHD ($N = 12$) with patients on CHD ($N = 22$). Three sets of QOL assessment tools were used. Patients on SDHD and NHD reported feeling better. They reported fewer and less severe cramping during dialysis, fewer headaches, fewer episodes of hypotension and dizziness, decreased fluid restrictions, decreased interdialytic weight gains, fewer episodes of shortness of breath, reduction in the sensation of easily feeling cold, and better maintenance of functionality compared to control patients on CHD.[17] The same year, McFarlane et al. compared QOL and costs and benefits between patients on NHD and on CHD. They showed that NHD was associated with a higher QOL scores and better cost utility compared to CHD.[18]

A Swedish study using the SF-36 health survey was done to demonstrate the effect of different dialysis modalities on QOL. Three groups of patients were studied: HHD patients ($N = 5$), a group of self-care patients who dialyze themselves in a center ($N = 6$), and CHD patients ($N = 8$). The QOL of patients on HHD was superior to the other two modalities. They further noted that self-care patients scored higher on several QOL parameters compared to CHD.[19] That was confirmed in a Japanese study showing better scores on seven out of eight QOL domains in HHD patients ($N = 46$) compared to CHD patients ($N = 34$).[20]

More recently, two review articles were published. Walker et al. reviewed 61 studies published between January 2000 and July 2016 that examined the patient-centered and economic impact of HHD. They showed that patients cared about several QOL parameters such as daytime freedom and flexibility, employment, fatigue, care partner burden, and ability to maintain normal activities. They further demonstrated that HHD offers the opportunity for a better QOL with improved freedom, flexibility, and well-being as well as strengthening family relationships.[21] Miller et al. carried out a systematic review of 44 publications to compare several outcome measures between HHD and CHD. Their review included seven publications that focused on QOL of both HHD and CHD patients. Compared to CHD, HHD-treated patients reported higher overall and specific component scores on standardized Hr-QOL.[22]

To assess changes in QOL on switching dialysis modalities, Vos et al. examined patients on CHD who switched to SDHD ($N = 13$). They obtained Hr-QOL, electroencephalogram (EEG), and neuropsychological assessment at baseline and 6 months after switching to SDHD. Patients were then switched back to CHD and the same studies were repeated 2 months later. The researchers showed that SDHD improved Hr-QOL with no clear effects on cognitive functioning and EEG. Resumption of CHD after SDHD decreased aspects of QOL with no effect on cognitive functioning.[23] Similar results were noted in a Chinese study by Jiang et al. which evaluated QOL in patients who switched from CHD to SDHD ($N = 27$). QOL was evaluated by SF-36 at baseline and 6 months after switching modality and showed an increase in the physical and mental health survey scores on the SDHD modality.[24] Furthermore, Jaber et al. showed that a switch in regimen from CHD to SDHD was associated with a 10-fold decrease in postdialysis recovery time and improved clinical depression.[25] Eneanya et al. retrospectively reviewed a national cohort study of adult patients to compare KDQOL-36 scores between CHD patients ($N = 4234$) and HHD patients ($N = 880$) and to examine the effect of switching modalities on the QOL. They showed that patients who switched from home to in-center dialysis ($N = 66$) had significantly lower physical functioning over time.[26]

While several studies have confirmed superior QOL in patients managed by SDHD over CHD, whether NHD affects QOL is unclear. The effect of NHD on QOL is more variable, depending on the cohort and assessment tool/scale used. Culleton et al. conducted a randomized, control trial comparing several parameters including QOL between patients on NHD ($N = 27$) and CHD ($N = 25$). While there were significant improvements in kidney-specific QOL domains and burden of kidney disease among NHD patients, there was no change noted in the global QOL as assessed by EuroQol 5-Dimension.[27] Furthermore, Rocco et al. showed no difference in physical health composite score between patients on NHD ($N = 45$) and CHD ($N = 42$), with both groups showing improved QOL.[28] Unruh et al. analyzed the results of the Frequent Hemodialysis Network (FHN) trials and showed no significant changes in self-reported depressive symptoms, mental health composite score, or emotional score among NHD and CHD patients.[29]

Quality of Life of Care Partners of Patients on Home Hemodialysis

Despite the recent approval by Food and Drug Administration (FDA) for solo HHD during a patient's waking hours, most of the patients on HHD depend on their care partners to assist with their dialysis as well as with their daily activities.[30] Care partners of HD patients endure significant pressure as a result of caring for patients with chronic illness, which can affect their QOL. It is likely that care partners for patients on HHD carry a heavier burden compared to those caring for patients undergoing CHD. Yet, fewer studies have been done to examine the QOL of care partners for HHD patients as compared to those for CHD patients.[31,32]

To compare the burden of care partners across dialysis modalities, Suri et al. examined the CHD care partner burden to that of non-paid NHD care partners ($N = 33$) and noted a trend of increased care partner burden among NHD care partners.[33] Gilbertson et al. expanded on this study and conducted a systematic review of quantitative studies of QOL and burden in care partners ($N = 5367$) of patients on different dialysis modalities: 72.3% CHD, 20.6% PD, and 7.1% HHD. Their results were different from the prior study, as they found that care partner QOL was comparable across dialysis modalities. Furthermore, they demonstrated that while QOL in dialysis patient care partners was poorer than in the general population, it was mostly comparable to QOL in care partners of people with other chronic diseases, and often better than QOL in the dialysis patients they cared for.[34]

Rioux et al. assessed the burden, QOL, and depressive symptoms in 31 NHD patients and their care partners. They showed that compared to their care partners, patients had lower perceived physical health scores and met more depression criteria but had similar mental health scores.[35] Walker et al. conducted a systemic review of 24 qualitative studies ($N =109$ patients and 121 care partners) that described patient and care partner perspectives and experiences with HHD. Although both patients and care partners had a more positive perspective on freedom, flexibility, and well-being compared to hospital dialysis patients, both groups had significant concerns. Patients verbalized their concerns about adding extra burden on their care partners, while care partners were concerned about being socially isolated with having less time to themselves, anxiety about being responsible of the medical needs of their loved ones, and the emotional strain they suffered from seeing their loved ones sick.[36] A year later, the same group underwent semi-structured interviews with 4 patients on HHD, as well as 40 patients who were predialysis ($N = 18$), on PD ($N = 13$) and CHD ($N = 9$). Nine care partners were also interviewed. They showed that care partners of dialysis patients reported that taking care of the patients was causing difficulty in sustaining relationships with their community and family, disrupting their lifestyle as well as resulting in feelings of letting down their other dependents, affecting their QOL negatively.[37]

▌CONCLUSION

HHD is a viable dialysis modality that is underused. While studies have shown that the QOL of patients on SDHD is superior to that of patients on CHD, data are controversial for patients on NHD. QOL of care partners of HHD patients can be negatively affected. Addressing concerns of both HHD patients and their care partners may help improve their QOL. Providers should consider patients' individual needs and expectations and offer respite care as well as social and emotional support to both patients and their care partners. Furthermore, routine evaluations of the QOL of care partners should be part of the monthly clinic visit.

▌REFERENCES

1. Sepucha KR, Fowler FJ Jr, Mulley AG Jr. Policy support for patient-centered care: the need for measurable improvements in decision quality. *Health Aff.* 2004;Suppl Variation:VAR54-62.
2. McFarlane P, Komenda P. Economic considerations in frequent home hemodialysis. *Semin Dialysis.* 2011;24(6):678-683.
3. Mapes DL, Lopes AA, Satayathum S, et al. Health-related quality of life as a predictor of mortality and hospitalization: the Dialysis Outcomes and Practice Patterns Study (DOPPS). *Kidney Int.* 2003;64:339-349.
4. Nagarathnam M, Sivakumar V, Latheef S. Burden, coping mechanisms, and quality of life among caregivers of hemodialysis and peritoneal dialysis undergoing and renal transplant patients. *Indian J Psychaitry.* 2019;61(4):380-388.
5. Bardak S, Demir S, Aslan E, et al. The other side of the coin in renal replacement therapies: the burden on caregivers. *Int Urol Nephrol.* 2019;51:343-349.
6. Lohr KN. Outcome measurement: concepts and questions. *Inquiry.* 1988;25(1):37-50.
7. Meyer KB, Espindle DM, DeGiacomo JM, et al. Monitoring dialysis patients' health status and its subset, the Short Form-12 Health Survey. *Am J Kidney Dis.* 1994;24:267-279.
8. Ware J Jr, Kosinski M, Keller SD. A 12-item Short Form Health Survey: construction of scales and preliminary tests of reliability and validity. *Med Care.* 1996;34:220-233.
9. Tomita K. Practice of home hemodialysis in dialysis clinic. *Contrib Nephrol.* 2012;177:143-150.
10. Piccoli GB, Bechis F, Iaczzo C, et al. Why our patients like daily dialysis. *Hemodial Int.* 2000;4(1):47-50.
11. Agar JW. International variations and trends in home hemodialysis. *Adv Chronic Kidney Dis.* 2009;16(3):205-214.
12. Susantitaphong P, Koulouridis I, Balk EM, et al. Effect of frequent or extended hemodialysis on cardiovascular parameters: a meta-analysis. *Am J Kidney Dis.* 2012;59(5):689-699.
13. Daugirdas JT, Chertow GM, Larive B, et al. Effects of frequent hemodialysis on measures of CKD mineral and bone disorders. *J Am Soc Nephrol.* 2012;23:727-738.
14. Karkar A, Hegbrant J, Strippoli GF. Benefits and implementation of home hemodialysis: a narrative review. *Saudi J Kidney Dis Transpl.* 2015;26:1095-1107.

15. Pauly RP, Gill JS, Rose CL, et al. Survival among nocturnal home hemodialysis patients compared to kidney transplant recipients. *Nephrol Dial Transplant.* 2009;24: 2915-2919.

16. Mohr PE, Neumann PJ, Franco SJ, et al. The case for daily dialysis: its impact on costs and quality of life. *Am J Kidney Dis.* 2011;37(4):777-789.

17. Heidenheim AP, Muirhead N, Moist L, et al. Patient quality of life on quotidian hemodialysis. *Am J Kidney Dis.* 2003;42(S1):S36-S41.

18. McFarlane PA, Bayoumi AM, Pierratos A, Redelmeier DA. The quality of life and cost utility of home nocturnal and conventional in-center hemodialysis. *Kidney Int.* 2003;64(3):1004-1011.

19. Ageborg M, Allenius B, Cederfjall C. Quality of life, self-care ability, and sense of coherence in hemodialysis patients: a comparative study. *Hemodial Int.* 2005; 9:S8-S14.

20. Watamabe Y, Ohno Y, Inoue T, et al. Home hemodialysis and conventional in-center hemodialysis in Japan: a comparison of health-related quality of life. *Hemodial Int.* 2014;18:S32-S38.

21. Walker RC, Howard K, Morton RL. Home hemodialysis: a comprehensive review of patient-centered and economic considerations. *Clinicoecon Outcomes Res.* 2017;9:149-161.

22. Miller BW, Himmele R, Sawin D, et al. Choosing home hemodialysis: a critical review of patient outcomes. *Blood Purif.* 2018;45:224-229.

23. Vos PF, Zilch O, Jennekens-Schinkel A. Effect of short daily home hemodialysis on quality of life, cognitive functioning and the electroencephalogram. *Nephrol Dial Transplant.* 2006;21:2529-2535.

24. Jiang JL, Ren W, Song J, et al. The impact of short daily hemodialysis on anemia and the quality of life in Chinese patients. *Braz J Med Biol Res.* 2013; 467(7):629-633.

25. Jaber BL, Lee Y, Collins AJ, et al. Effect of daily hemodialysis on depressive symptoms and post-dialysis recovery time: interim report from the FREEDOM (Following Rehabilitation, Economics and Everyday Dialysis Outcome Measurements) study. *Am J Kidney Dis.* 2010;56(3):531-539.

26. Eneanya ND, Maddux DW, Reviriego-Mendoza MM, et al. Longitudinal patterns of health-related quality of life and dialysis modality: a national cohort study. *BMC Nephrol.* 2019;20:7.

27. Culleton BF, Walsh M, Klarenbach SW, et al. Effect of frequent nocturnal hemodialysis vs conventional hemodialysis on left ventricular mass and quality of life: a randomized controlled trial. *JAMA.* 2007;298:1291-1299.

28. Rocco MV, Lockridge RS Jr, Beck GJ, et al. The effects of frequent nocturnal home hemodialysis: the frequent hemodialysis network nocturnal trial. *Kidney Int.* 2011;80:1080-1091.

29. Unruh ML, Larive B, Chertow GM. Effects of 6-times-weekly versus 3-times-weekly hemodialysis on depressive symptoms and self-reported mental health: Frequent Hemodialysis Network (FHN) trials. *Am J Kidney Dis.* 2013; 61(5):748-758.

30. Food and Drug Administration, US Department of Health and Human Services. NxStage System One: Section 510(k) premarket notification. Silver Spring, MD: Food and Drug Administration; 2017.

31. Nagasawa H, Sugita I, Tachi T, et al. The relationship between dialysis patients' quality of life and caregivers' quality of life. *Front Pharmacol.* 2018;9:1-10.

32. Jafari H, Ebrahimi A, Aghaei A, et al. The relationship between care burden and quality of life in caregivers of hemodialysis patients. *BMC Nephrol.* 2018;19:321.

33. Suri RS, Larive B, Hall Y, et al. Effects of frequent hemodialysis on perceived caregiver burden in the Frequent Hemodialysis Network trials. *Clin J Am Soc Nephrol.* 2014;9(5):936-942.

34. Gilbertson EL, Krishnasamy R, Foote C, et al. Burden of care and quality of life among caregivers for adults receiving maintenance dialysis: a systematic review. *Am J Kidney Dis.* 2019;73(3):332-343.

35. Rioux J, Narayanan R, Chan C. Caregiver burden among nocturnal home hemodialysis patients. *Hemodial Int.* 2012;16:214-219.

36. Walker RC, Morton RL, Tong A, et al. Patient and caregiver values, beliefs and experiences when considering home dialysis as a treatment option: a semi-structured interview study. *Nephrol Dial Transplant.* 2016;31:133-141.

37. Walker RC, Hanson CS, Palmer SC, et al. Patient and caregiver perspectives on home hemodialysis: a systematic review. *Am J Kidney Dis.* 2015;65(3):451-463.

12 HOSPITALIZATION AND HOME HEMODIALYSIS

Eric Weinhandl

Hospitalization remains one of the greatest burdens in the dialysis patient population. According to the United States Renal Data System (USRDS), the rate of hospital admission in dialysis patients with Medicare fee-for-service coverage during 2017 was 1750 admissions per 1000 patient-years. Although this rate of hospital admissions is modestly lower than the corresponding rate 15 years earlier, it has exhibited little movement during the most recent 5 years of data collection. With respect to cumulative duration of hospitalization, the rate of hospitalized days in dialysis patients with Medicare fee-for-service coverage in 2017 was 11.2 days per patient-year. Interestingly, this rate translates to roughly 45 hospitalized minutes per calendar day. From that perspective, the human toll of hospitalization on dialysis patients and their families is plainly evident.[1]

The human toll is rivaled by the economic toll. Again, according to the USRDS, cumulative Medicare Parts A, B, and D expenditures among dialysis patients with Medicare coverage during 2017 was $90,549 per patient-year. Of this total, $27,517 were attributable to inpatient facility payments and $3207 were attributable to physician payments in in-patient settings. Furthermore, another $3482 were attributed to skilled nursing facility payments, which are almost always subsequent to hospital discharge.[1] Therefore, between 35% and 40% of all Medicare spending in the dialysis patient population is connected to hospitalization and post-acute care. As the cost of outpatient dialysis treatment is relatively fixed on a per-annum basis, it is clear that any serious attempt at reducing spending in the dialysis patient population begins—and possibly ends— with efforts aimed at lower hospitalization risk.

Whether home hemodialysis (HHD) can alter hospitalization risk remains fundamentally unclear. Of course, the dominant prescriptions of HHD vary from one country to another. In New Zealand, Australia, and Canada, where HHD constitutes a larger share of the dialytic modality mix than in the United States, thrice-weekly treatment is common.[1–3] In both Australia and New Zealand, roughly half of HHD patients dialyze three times per week. However, only 20% of HHD patients in Australia and New Zealand accumulate less than 15 hours of treatment per week.[4] Thus, HHD is characterized by an increase in the cumulative duration of treatment, even when the frequency of treatment is unaltered. Extending the duration of treatment clearly lowers the ultrafiltration rate and likely increases the total removal of middle molecules, but if the frequency of treatment is unaltered, the long interdialytic gap and its associated morbidity may be unaddressed.[5,6] This may have important consequences for hospitalization risk. In the United States, the contemporary application of HHD is dominated by low-flow dialysate, so HHD and frequent hemodialysis (HD) (i.e., treatment for >3 sessions per week) are tightly connected.[7] On the other hand, utilization of nocturnal hemodialysis (NHD) has greatly lagged utilization of diurnal HD. In the home setting, diurnal HD typically involves four, five, or six treatments per week, at a duration between 150 and 200 minutes per session. Thus, HHD in the United States is characterized by an increase in the frequency of treatment, but not necessarily a substantial increase in the cumulative duration of treatment. Increasing the frequency of treatment is likely to eliminate the long interdialytic gap, but if the cumulative duration of treatment is unaltered, the total removal of solutes whose clearance is time-dependent may be unchanged, relative to thrice-weekly in-center HD. This, too, may have important consequences for hospitalization risk.

Complicating matters is the self-evident setting of HHD: the home. Patients who select HD in the home setting may have substantially different demographic and clinical characteristics than those patients who select HD in the facility setting. Unfortunately, the literature does not include a randomized clinical trial of home versus in-center HD, given fixed frequency and duration of treatment. It is highly likely that no such trial will ever be feasible. Therefore, the causal effect of home versus in-center HD on hospitalization risk will remain unknown. Nevertheless, the literature is populated with non-randomized studies that estimate the association of home versus in-center HD with hospitalization risk. Because these studies are observational, they may be subject to unmeasured confounding, especially if HHD patients tend to be healthier than their counterparts who dialyze in the facility setting. Overall, these studies provide a window into the major sources of morbidity that HHD patients experience, including sources that may be either more or less likely to manifest in the home setting, relative to the facility setting.

DAILY HOME HEMODIALYSIS AND HOSPITALIZATION RISK IN THE UNITED STATES

The most comprehensive study of hospitalization risk in HHD patients was reported by Weinhandl et al.[8] The study included 3480 patients who initiated HHD with the NxStage System One between January 1, 2006, and December 31, 2009. All patients were initially prescribed either five or six treatments per week; nearly 95% of patients during that era were prescribed either five or six treatments per week, so the winnowing effect of this inclusion criterion was not strong. However, all patients were also required to carry Medicare Parts A and B as primary payer. Only 60% of HHD patients during that era carried Medicare Parts A and B as the primary payer; to this day, very little is known about hospitalization risk in HHD patients with other classes of health insurance, including Medicare Advantage and private insurance.[8]

The study included a comparator group of matched in-center HD patients with Medicare fee-for-service coverage. For each patient undergoing HHD, the study investigators selected five matched controls from a large pool of candidate controls. Each candidate control underwent in-center HD on the same calendar date on which the HHD patient began HD in the home setting. Matched controls were selected on the basis of an estimated propensity score of HHD initiation. That propensity score was a function of a wide array of factors, including age, race, sex, the primary cause of end-stage kidney disease (ESKD), the cumulative duration of ESKD (i.e., at the initiation of follow-up), concurrent enrollment in Medicare and Medicaid, comorbid conditions, body mass index, hospitalization history, kidney transplant wait-list registration, and dialysis provider organization. The set of comorbid conditions comprised 7 cardiovascular conditions and 11 non-cardiovascular conditions. Because of this methodology, the study was rigorously adjusted for measured factors. However, unmeasured factors, including biochemistry and frailty, may have contributed to the reported associations of dialytic modality with hospitalization risk.[8]

Patients were followed until the earliest of death, kidney transplantation, loss of Medicare Parts A and B as primary payer, and either December 31, 2009 (among patients whose follow-up began in 2006 or 2007), or December 31, 2010 (among patients whose follow-up began in 2008 or 2009). This follow-up rule was akin to an intention-to-treat analysis, insofar as patients were followed beyond any change in dialytic modality. In a sensitivity analysis, the study investigators added change in dialytic modality to the follow-up rule. However, results were unchanged.[8]

The study assessed not only rates of all-cause hospital admissions and hospitalized days, but also rates of cause-specific hospital admissions. Causes of hospitalization were defined according to the principal discharge diagnosis. Broad categories comprised cardiovascular morbidity, infection, vascular access dysfunction (i.e., morbidity excluding infection of the vascular access), and other morbidity. Within the broad category of cardiovascular morbidity, finer categories of hospitalization comprised arrhythmia; cerebrovascular disease; heart failure, fluid overload, and cardiomyopathy; hypertensive disease; ischemic heart disease; and other cardiovascular morbidity. Within the broad category of infection, finer categories of hospitalization comprised bacteremia and sepsis; cardiac infection; human immunodeficiency virus; osteomyelitis; respiratory infection; urinary tract infection; vascular access infection; and other infection.[8]

In the intention-to-treat analysis, the cumulative incidence of hospitalization at 1 year was 63% and 58% in HHD and matched in-center HD patients, respectively; at 2 years, corresponding estimates of cumulative incidence were 80% and 75%. Thus, the majority of patients on HHD were hospitalized during the first 2 years of treatment and the cumulative incidence of hospitalization with HHD appeared to be no lower than with in-center HD. Indeed, the hazard ratios of all-cause hospitalization with HHD versus in-center HD were 1.03 (95% confidence interval, 0.99 to 1.08) in intention-to-treat analysis and 1.04 (0.98 to 1.11) in on-treatment analysis.[8]

However, the apparent neutrality in all-cause hospitalization obscures tremendous detail in cause-specific hospitalization. First, the hazard ratios of cardiovascular-related hospitalization with HHD versus in-center HD were 0.83 (0.78 to 0.88) in intention-to-treat analysis and 0.77 (0.72 to 0.82) in on-treatment analysis. Conversely, the hazard ratios of infection-related hospitalization were 1.32 (1.24 to 1.40) in intention-to-treat analysis and 1.30 (1.22 to 1.39) in on-treatment analysis. Thus, HHD patients were less likely to be hospitalized for cardiovascular morbidity than in-center HD patients were, but HHD patients were more likely to be hospitalized for infection-related morbidity. These causes of hospitalization were responsible for slightly more than half of all hospitalizations. Associations of dialytic modality with risks of hospitalization for vascular access dysfunction and other morbidity were very weak.[8]

Regarding cardiovascular morbidity, hazard ratios of cause-specific hospitalization with HHD versus in-center HD were 0.97 (0.84 to 1.12) for arrhythmia; 0.85 (0.71 to 1.02) for cerebrovascular disease; 0.69 (0.62 to 0.77) for heart failure, fluid overload, and cardiomyopathy; 0.88 (0.80 to 0.96) for hypertensive disease; 0.94 (0.84 to 1.05) for ischemic heart disease; 1.06 (0.95 to 1.18) for peripheral arterial disease; and 1.18 (0.98 to 1.41) for other cardiovascular morbidity. The categories of cerebrovascular disease, heart failure, and hypertensive disease together constituted about half of all cardiovascular-related hospitalizations. That HHD patients had lower risks of hospitalization in each of these categories likely reflects the effects of increased frequency of treatment. As the Frequent Hemodialysis Network (FHN) Daily Trial showed, frequent HD lowers blood pressure and decreases ultrafiltration volume per treatment.[9,10] Furthermore, frequent HD decreases left ventricular mass.[9,11] Thus, it seems reasonable to conclude that frequent HHD likely lowers the risk of cardiovascular morbidity that is sensitive to volume and pressure load. From that perspective, it is also interesting that HHD patients did not have lower risk of hospitalization due to arrhythmia. During the study era, most HHD patients used dialysate that included 1 mmol/L of potassium. The difference in predialysis serum potassium and dialysate potassium concentrations may have been sufficiently large to be arrhythmogenic. This area requires further investigation.

Regarding infection, hazard ratios of cause-specific hospitalization with HHD versus in-center HD were 1.35 (1.24 to 1.46) for bacteremia and sepsis; 3.42 (2.57 to 4.55) for cardiac infection; 0.94 (0.65 to 1.37) for human immunodeficiency virus; 1.48 (1.14 to 1.93) for osteomyelitis; 0.94 (0.86 to 1.03) for respiratory infection; 1.01 (0.79 to 1.29) for urinary tract infection; 1.39 (1.28 to 1.50) for vascular access infection; and 1.22 (1.12 to 1.31) for other infection. The categories of bacteremia and sepsis and vascular access infection together constituted nearly half of all infection-related hospitalizations, whereas the categories of cardiac infection and osteomyelitis—both metastatic infections—together constituted slightly more than 5% of all infection-related hospitalizations. Interestingly, the hazard ratios of first infection-related hospitalization and recurrent infection-related hospitalizations (in patients with a first infection-related hospitalization) were 1.35 and 1.03, respectively. This discrepancy indicates that HHD patients were more likely than in-center HD patients to experience a first infection-related hospitalization, but after discharge, HHD patients were not more likely than in-center HD patients to be hospitalized again for infection. This discrepancy suggests that frequency is an unlikely explanation for the association of HHD with higher risk of infection-related hospitalization and instead points to gaps in cannulation technique and infection control.

Buttonhole cannulation, which is relatively popular among HHD patients, may be a culprit.[12] One systematic review reported that in randomized clinical trials and observational studies, relative risks of fistula-related infection with buttonhole versus rope-ladder cannulation were 3.34 and 3.15, respectively.[13] Other studies have found that buttonhole cannulation is associated with increased incidence of infections with metastatic complications, such as infective endocarditis.[14] On the other hand, interventional studies have reported that the risk of infection with buttonhole cannulation may be mitigated by the prophylactic use of mupirocin ointment.[15] An alternative explanation is that HHD patients experience delayed diagnosis and treatment of vascular access infection. In this scenario, the incidence of vascular access infection in the outpatient setting might be similar with HHD and in-center HD, but because of delays in diagnosis and treatment, infection-related hospitalization is more likely on HHD. In any case, a survey of practices in 19 HHD training centers found that nurses were not instructing HHD patients in generally accepted practices and patients were not cannulating according to generally accepted practices.[16] Thus, lowering hospitalization risk on HHD probably requires greater attention to cannulation technique and infection control.

HOSPITALIZATION RISK WITH HOME HEMODIALYSIS VERSUS PERITONEAL DIALYSIS

There have been two observational studies that have compared hospitalization risk with HHD and peritoneal dialysis (PD). The comparison of hospitalization risk with HHD versus PD is insightful, as both modalities are situated in the home setting, thus eliminating the potential for confounding inherent in the contrast between home and in-center HD. However, the comparison of hospitalization risk with HHD versus PD is complicated by the fact that most PD patients initiate treatment with the modality at or shortly after dialysis initiation, whereas most HHD patients initiate treatment with the modality years after dialysis initiation.

Suri et al. compared the hospitalization risk of 1116 HHD patients in a large dialysis organization with the corresponding risk of 2784 matched PD patients in the same dialysis organization.[17] Patients were matched according to a propensity score of HHD, itself a function of age, race, sex, duration of ESKD, eight comorbid conditions, body mass index, smoking status, serum albumin, and hemoglobin. The hazard ratio of all-cause hospitalization with HHD versus PD was 0.73 (0.67 to 0.79). The hazard ratios of cardiac and infection-related hospitalization with HHD versus PD were 0.66 (0.58 to 0.74) and 0.81 (0.73 to 0.90). Thus, HHD was generally associated with lower risk of hospitalization, relative to PD.

Weinhandl et al. compared the hospitalization risk of 3301 HHD patients with the corresponding risk of 3301 matched PD patients.[18] All HHD patients used the NxStage System One, were prescribed either five or six treatments per week, and carried Medicare Parts A and B as primary payer. All PD patients likewise carried Medicare Parts A and B as primary payer; these patients may have utilized either continuous ambulatory or cycler-assisted PD. Patients were matched according to a propensity score of HHD, itself a function of age, race, sex, the primary cause of ESKD, the duration of ESKD, concurrent enrollment in Medicare and Medicaid, enrollment in Medicare Part D, comorbid conditions, body mass index, hospitalization history, kidney transplant wait-list registration, dialysis provider organization, and in patients who initiated dialysis, both estimated glomerular filtration rate and hemoglobin at dialysis initiation.

The hazard ratio of all-cause hospitalization with HHD versus PD was 0.85 (0.89 to 0.95). The hazard ratio of cardiovascular-related hospitalization with HHD versus PD was 0.85 (0.80 to 0.91), whereas the hazard ratio of infection-related hospitalization with HHD versus PD was 0.89 (0.84 to 0.94). Interestingly, the relative rate of all-cause hospitalized days with HHD versus PD was 0.81 (0.75 to 0.87), thereby suggesting that length of stay for hospitalized HHD patients was generally shorter than length of stay for hospitalized PD patients. This suggestion was especially evident in the case of cardiovascular-related hospitalization.

In a sensitivity analysis, only the subset of 468 HHD patients and 468 matched PD patients who initiated home dialysis within 6 months after the diagnosis of ESKD were retained for analysis. In this subset, the hazard ratio of all-cause hospitalization with HHD versus PD was 0.96 (0.88 to 1.05). The hazard ratio of cardiovascular-related hospitalization with HHD versus PD was 0.89 (0.75 to 1.06), whereas the hazard ratio of infection-related hospitalization with HHD versus PD was 1.01 (0.87 to 1.18). The lack of statistical significance in any of these associations may reflect the limited sample size in this analysis, or alternatively, may reflect that hospitalization risks with HHD and PD are very similar during the first years of ESKD.

HOSPITALIZATION RISK WITH HOME HEMODIALYSIS VERSUS KIDNEY TRANSPLANTATION

Tennankore et al. reported hospitalization risk in 173 patients who underwent intensive HHD (i.e., cumulative duration of treatment equal to or greater than 16 hours per week) and patients who received a kidney transplant.[19] The latter group of patients were stratified into 673 patients who received a living donor transplant, 642 patients who received a deceased donor transplant of standard criteria, and 202 patients who received a deceased donor transplant of extended criteria. In an adjusted model, hospitalization risk in all strata of kidney transplant recipients was between 15 and 19 times higher during the first month after transplantation, relative to the first month of HHD, and between 5 and 8 times higher during the second and third months after transplantation, relative to the second and third months of HHD. Conversely, after the first year of follow-up, the relative rate of hospitalization for living donor transplantation versus intensive HHD was 0.64 (0.47 to 0.87). However, the relative rate of hospitalization for deceased donor transplantation of standard criteria versus intensive HHD was 0.96 (0.69 to 1.34) and for deceased donor transplantation of extended criteria versus intensive HHD was 0.80 (0.54 to 1.19). Thus, intensive HHD is associated with similar long-term risk of hospitalization as kidney transplantation with a deceased donor.

EVIDENCE FROM RANDOMIZED CLINICAL TRIALS

The FHN Nocturnal Trial and an earlier randomized trial in Alberta both tested the effects of frequent NHD versus thrice-weekly HD in the home setting.[20,21] The FHN Nocturnal Trial included 87 patients and the earlier trial in Alberta included only 51 patients. Thus, both trials were clearly underpowered to assess the effects of frequent on hospitalization risk in the home setting. In the FHN Nocturnal Trial, there were 43 hospitalizations among 19 of 45 patients on NHD and 30 hospitalizations among 16 of 42 patients on conventional HD. The hazard ratio of all-cause hospitalization with nocturnal versus conventional HD was 1.62 (0.91 to 2.87). On the other hand, in the earlier trial in Alberta, there were 0.62 hospitalizations per patient with NHD and 0.84

hospitalizations per patient with conventional HD. Thus, trial evidence offers conflicting signals about the effect of HD frequency on hospitalization risk in the home setting.

▌GAPS IN KNOWLEDGE

Much about hospitalization with HHD remains to be studied. First, there is very sparse literature about the hospitalization of HHD patients outside of the United States. The clearest consequence of this gap in knowledge is uncertainty about hospitalization risk associated with nocturnal versus diurnal HD, regardless of the frequency of treatment. One study of 32 Canadian patients who underwent nocturnal HHD suggested that conversion from conventional in-center HD to nocturnal HHD was associated with a sharp decline in cardiovascular-related hospitalization risk, relative to matched control patients who remained on conventional in-center HD, but the association was only nominally significant ($P = 0.04$).[22]

Second, there are no large studies of 30-day readmission risk with HHD versus other dialytic modalities. In addition, there has recently been a shift in acute care from inpatient to outpatient settings, as exemplified by observation status admissions and emergency department visits. No published study has characterized acute care of HHD patients in the outpatient setting.

Third, there is no literature about the nature of dialysis during the hospitalization of an HHD patient. It is unclear whether frequent HD is discontinued during hospitalization. When patients are discharged, especially to a skilled nursing facility for post-acute care, it is unclear whether there manifests temporarily increased risk of HHD technique failure.

Fourth, and perhaps surprisingly, the literature about risk factors for hospitalization on HHD is underdeveloped. A recent study suggested that standardized Kt/V was not significantly associated with risk of hospitalization.[23] Another study of 165 patients in a regional dialysis provider organization found that intensity of HHD was not associated with infection-related hospitalization risk.[24]

▌REFERENCES

1. Saran R, Robinson B, Abbott KC, et al. US Renal Data System 2019 Annual Data Report: epidemiology of kidney disease in the United States. *Am J Kidney Dis*. 2020;75(1S1):A6-A7.
2. ANZDATA Registry. 41st Report, Chapter 2: prevalence of end stage kidney disease. Australia and New Zealand Dialysis and Transplant Registry, Adelaide,

Australia. 2018. Available at http://www.anzdata.org.au. Accessed January 15, 2020.

3. Canadian Institute for Health Information. Treatment of end-stage organ failure in Canada, Canadian Organ Replacement Register, 2009 to 2018: end-stage kidney disease and kidney transplants—data tables. 2019.

4. ANZDATA Registry. 41st Report, Chapter 4: haemodialysis. Australia and New Zealand Dialysis and Transplant Registry, Adelaide, Australia. 2018. Available at http://www.anzdata.org.au. Accessed January 15, 2020.

5. Raj DS, Ouwendyk M, Francoeur R, Pierratos A. beta(2)-microglobulin kinetics in nocturnal haemodialysis. *Nephrol Dial Transplant*. 2000;15(1):58-64.

6. Foley RN, Gilbertson DT, Murray T, Collins AJ. Long interdialytic interval and mortality among patients receiving hemodialysis. *N Engl J Med*. 2011;365(12):1099-1107.

7. Lockridge R, Cornelis T, Van Eps C. Prescriptions for home hemodialysis. *Hemodial Int*. 2015;19(suppl 1):S112-S127.

8. Weinhandl ED, Nieman KM, Gilbertson DT, Collins AJ. Hospitalization in daily home hemodialysis and matched thrice-weekly in-center hemodialysis patients. *Am J Kidney Dis*. 2015;65(1):98-108.

9. FHN Trial Group, Chertow GM, Levin NW, et al. In-center hemodialysis six times per week versus three times per week. *N Engl J Med*. 2010;363(24):2287-2300.

10. Kotanko P, Garg AX, Depner T, et al. Effects of frequent hemodialysis on blood pressure: results from the randomized frequent hemodialysis network trials. *Hemodial Int*. 2015;19(3):386-401.

11. Chan CT, Greene T, Chertow GM, et al. Determinants of left ventricular mass in patients on hemodialysis: Frequent Hemodialysis Network (FHN) trials. *Circ Cardiovasc Imaging*. 2012;5(2):251-261.

12. Faratro R, Jeffries J, Nesrallah GE, MacRae JM. The care and keeping of vascular access for home hemodialysis patients. *Hemodial Int*. 2015;19(suppl 1):S80-S92.

13. Muir CA, Kotwal SS, Hawley CM, et al. Buttonhole cannulation and clinical outcomes in a home hemodialysis cohort and systematic review. *Clin J Am Soc Nephrol*. 2014;9(1):110-119.

14. Wong B, Muneer M, Wiebe N, et al. Buttonhole versus rope-ladder cannulation of arteriovenous fistulas for hemodialysis: a systematic review. *Am J Kidney Dis*. 2014;64(6):918-936.

15. Nesrallah GE, Cuerden M, Wong JHS, Pierratos A. *Staphylococcus aureus* bacteremia and buttonhole cannulation: long-term safety and efficacy of mupirocin prophylaxis. *Clin J Am Soc Nephrol*. 2010;5(6):1047-1053.

16. Spry LA, Burkart JM, Holcroft C, Mortier L, Glickman JD. Survey of home hemodialysis patients and nursing staff regarding vascular access use and care. *Hemodial Int*. 2015;19(2):225-234.

17. Suri RS, Li L, Nesrallah GE. The risk of hospitalization and modality failure with home dialysis. *Kidney Int*. 2015;88(2):360-368.

18. Weinhandl ED, Gilbertson DT, Collins AJ. Mortality, hospitalization, and technique failure in daily home hemodialysis and matched peritoneal dialysis patients: a matched cohort study. *Am J Kidney Dis*. 2016;67(1):98-110.

19. Tennankore KK, Kim SJ, Baer HJ, Chan CT. Survival and hospitalization for intensive home hemodialysis compared with kidney transplantation. *J Am Soc Nephrol*. 2014;25(9):2113-2120.

20. Rocco MV, Lockridge RS, Beck GJ, et al. The effects of frequent nocturnal home hemodialysis: the Frequent Hemodialysis Network Nocturnal Trial. *Kidney Int*. 2011;80(10):1080-1091.

21. Culleton BF, Walsh M, Klarenbach SW, et al. Effect of frequent nocturnal hemodialysis vs conventional hemodialysis on left ventricular mass and quality of life: a randomized controlled trial. *JAMA*. 2007;298(11):1291-1299.

22. Bergman A, Fenton SSA, Richardson RMA, Chan CT. Reduction in cardiovascular related hospitalization with nocturnal home hemodialysis. *Clin Nephrol*. 2008;69(1):33-39.

23. Rivara MB, Ravel V, Streja E, et al. Weekly standard Kt/Vurea and clinical outcomes in home and in-center hemodialysis. *Clin J Am Soc Nephrol*. 2018;13(3):445-455.

24. Bi S-H, Tang W, Rigodanzo-Massey N, et al. Infection-related hospitalizations in home hemodialysis patients. *Blood Purif*. 2015;40(3):187-193.

SPECIAL POPULATIONS AND HOME HEMODIALYSIS

13

Christopher T. Chan and Michael Girsberger

Home hemodialysis (HHD) and more frequent (or intensive) HHD have several advantages over thrice-weekly in-center hemodialysis (conventional hemodialysis [CHD]).[1] Certain patient populations have specific medical indications for intensive hemodialysis (HD) dosing (>12 hours of HD per week), and HHD provides the flexibility to tailor the HD prescription to the patient's needs. The aim of this chapter is to discuss specific patient populations that may benefit from more intense HD at home.

CARDIOVASCULAR INDICATIONS FOR INTENSIVE HEMODIALYSIS AT HOME

Patients with end-stage kidney disease (ESKD) have much higher cardiovascular mortality rates than the general population. In fact, according to the United States Renal Data System (USRDS), younger patients (40 to 44 years) started on CHD have a strikingly short average lifespan of only 8 years.[2] More frequent HHD has been shown to reverse left ventricular hypertrophy (LVH), improve blood pressure control, augment endothelial dependent vasodilatation, and restore nocturnal heart rate variability.[3] Additionally, more frequent HHD in the form of nocturnal hemodialysis (NHD) has been shown to normalize phosphorus levels and lower total peripheral resistance.[4,5] Taken together, patients who have increased cardiovascular burden (e.g., refractory hypertension [HTN] and LVH) should consider intensive HD as a unique therapeutic option.[6]

[For more information, see Chapters 7 and 9.]

Resistant Hypertension

Reaching euvolemia and normalizing blood pressure remains a common challenge in patients on CHD. Up to 80% of patients on HD have been reported to be hypertensive.[7] Salt and extracellular volume overload are highly prevalent in patients with chronic kidney disease (CKD) even prior to reaching ESKD. Enhanced filling pressure leads to increased cardiac output via the Frank-Starling mechanism, thereby elevating arterial pressure. Elevated total peripheral resistance has also been described previously as occurring through the following mechanisms[8]:

1. Decreased bioavailability of vasodilatory mediators such as nitric oxide in the uremic environment,
2. Increased arterial stiffness facilitated by vascular calcification, and
3. Elevations in vasoconstrictors such as angiotensin II and norepinephrine.

Better blood pressure control is one of the most consistent findings in more frequent HHD, which obviates the need for removal of large volumes in a short time. Up to 75% of patients had normal blood pressure while on short daily HHD in one study.[9] Interestingly, while improved blood pressure has been reported in both modalities (nocturnal and short daily HHD), the mechanisms leading to these findings may be different. In short daily HHD, patients saw a significant decrease in extracellular volume, suggesting that improved volume control was the main reason for lower blood pressure. In contrast, blood pressure decreased in nocturnal HHD despite the nadir of extracellular volume remaining unchanged. In this study, brachial artery responsiveness improved after 2 months on nocturnal HHD, indicative of reduced peripheral resistance.[5] Potential mechanisms for decreased peripheral vascular resistance in nocturnal HHD include restoration of vascular smooth muscle cell biology with improved vasodilatory capacity, reduction of sympathomimetic stimuli possibly due to better clearance of vasoconstrictive mediators, and improvement in sleep disorders such as obstructive sleep apnea (OSA).[10–12] It is important to note that many of these studies have been conducted in patients using standard HD machines. Whether these results are also applicable for those using low-flow HD machines (e.g., NxStage) remains to be investigated.

[For more information, see Chapter 7.]

Left Ventricular Hypertrophy and Impaired Left Ventricular Ejection Fraction

LVH occurs in patients with ESKD as a consequence of recurrent volume and pressure overload.[13] Indeed, LVH has been a consistent surrogate marker of cardiovascular mortality in most observational cohort and registry studies.[14,15] To date, more frequent HD in the form of short daily hemodialysis (SDHD) and NHD has been shown to improve LVH.[6] In the Frequent Hemodialysis Network (FHN) trials and the Alberta Kidney Network trial, intensive HD reduced LVH by 13.4 g within 6 to 12 months of initiating the modality (Table 13-1).[16] Baseline left ventricular mass (LVM) was consistently one of the most important determinants of the magnitude of reduction of LVM in the frequent HD group.[17] In nocturnal HHD, regression of LVH has also been shown to translate to better clinical outcomes.[18]

Reduced left ventricular ejection fraction (LVEF) poses a unique challenge in patients with ESKD. Patients with reduced LVEF are more susceptible to variations in extracellular volume and develop pulmonary edema and heart failure (HF) when volume overloaded. However, high ultrafiltration (UF) rates lead to recurrent hypotension and cardiac stunning, further deteriorating cardiac function. Impaired relaxation of the left ventricle and increased filling pressures contribute to further deterioration of left ventricular function. However, data on the effect of intensified HD on LVEF is sparse. In a study by Chan et al., six patients with severely reduced LVEF (mean 28%) who received intensified HD saw a sustained increase in LVEF.[19]

[For more information, see Chapters 7 and 9.]

Table 13-1 CHANGES IN LEFT VENTRICULAR PARAMETERS WITH INTENSIVE HEMODIALYSIS		
Parameter	Number of Studies	Effect Size
Left ventricular mass index (g/m^2)	23 studies, 524 patients	−31.2 (−39.8 to −22.5)
Left ventricular mass (g)	13 studies, 335 patients	−60.5 (−90.8 to −30.2)
Left ventricular mass (g) [in RCTs only]	3 studies	−13.4 (−19.5 to −7.4)
Left ventricular ejection fraction (%)	4 studies, 137 patients	6.7 (1.6 to 11.9)

Adapted from findings in Susantitaphong P, Koulouridis I, Balk EM, et al. Effect of frequent or extended hemodialysis on cardiovascular parameters: A meta-analysis. *Am J Kidney Dis*. 2012;59(5):689-699.

Pulmonary Hypertension

Right ventricular dysfunction and pulmonary HTN are both very common in ESKD. Pulmonary HTN has been reported in up to 50% of patients receiving CHD.[20] Increasing HD dose may modify endothelial cell biology and improve average extracellular volume control, potentially leading to improvement in right ventricular function and pulmonary HTN.[21] Overall, published literature on the effects of more frequent HHD on the right heart is scarce. Studies have shown improvement in right ventricular parameters in patients undergoing SDHD or NHD.[22] As for pulmonary HTN, only anecdotal literature has been published so far. We reported reduction of right ventricular systolic pressure and increase in clinical well-being in a patient with severe pulmonary HTN after initiating more frequent HHD.[23]

▌REFRACTORY HYPERPHOSPHATEMIA

Hyperphosphatemia is common in patients with ESKD. Reduced phosphate clearance induces fibroblast growth factor 23 (FGF-23), which inhibits hydroxylation of 25(OH) vitamin D to its active form 1, 25(OH) vitamin D. Propagation of chronic hyperphosphatemia and its systemic effects are part of the CKD-mineral bone disorder syndrome.[24]

Intensifying HD is an effective option to lower serum phosphate.[25] Phosphate is a relatively large molecule; therefore, clearance is time-dependent. Weekly clearance of phosphate with CHD ranges between 1500 and 3000 mg, but intake has been reported to be as high as 1500 mg daily. This explains why up to 30% of patients on CHD have persistent hyperphosphatemia despite adherence to phosphate binders. This is in stark contrast to more intense HD prescriptions. SDHD and NHD have been shown to reduce phosphate levels within a month of intensifying HD.[26,27] In fact, NHD is effective to such an extent that up to 40% of patients may require addition of phosphorus to their dialysate to prevent hypophosphatemia. Consequently, the prevalence of phosphate binder use decreased to less than 30% in these studies—even as low as zero in one study.[28] Reduction in use of phosphate binders not only reduces the patients' pill burden, but also reduces overall costs associated with ESKD care.

Whether more frequent HHD has any impact on parathyroid hormone (PTH) levels is unclear. Some studies have shown significant reduction in PTH after intensifying HD prescription, while others have not. Overall, secondary hyperparathyroidism (HPT) remains relatively unchanged with intensive HD. Most studies have focused on changes in laboratory parameters—studies of the clinical effects of these changes are very limited. In fact, only one study reported reduction of vascular calcification after initiation of SDHD.[29] Vascular calcification assessed with radiography was significantly lower in hands and feet after 12 months; no change was observed for aortic valve calcification. Overall, phosphate clearance can be significantly increased with more frequent HHD, which is an attractive option for patients with resistant hyperphosphatemia and secondary HPT. While improvement of hyperphosphatemia is well documented, there is paucity on studies on the clinical effect of these changes.

[For more information, see Chapters 7 and 10.]

∎ PATIENTS WITH SLEEP DISORDERS

Excessive daytime sleepiness and sleep disorders such as OSA, central sleep apnea, restless legs syndrome, and periodic leg movement may affect up to 50% of patients with ESKD.[30] Potential mechanisms include retention of uremic toxins and rostral fluid shift secondary to volume overload.[30–32]

Excessive daytime sleepiness has been mainly attributed to changes in sleep architecture with short and fragmented sleep, long wake times, and arousals along with day/night sleep reversal.[33] Inflammatory cytokine release during HD, reduced clearance of melatonin, and subclinical uremic encephalopathy have been proposed as pathophysiological mechanisms. An interesting study suggested arousals during sleep are caused by changes in amino acid metabolism; therefore, lower neurotransmitter activity may reduce sleep quality and contribute to excessive daytime sleepiness.[34] In fact, an experimental study showed improved sleep patterns after infusion of branched chain amino acids, further supporting this hypothesis.[35] These pathologic mechanisms may also be responsible for the higher prevalence of central sleep apnea and restless legs syndrome in ESKD.

Upper airway edema due to volume overload has been shown to cause or exacerbate OSA. Mechanistic studies have been conducted in patients on CHD as well as peritoneal dialysis (PD) implicating the causal role of rostral shifting of excess retained extracellular fluid, without modification of uremic clearance.[36] Several studies have investigated the effect of intensive HD on sleep disturbances. The most compelling of these by Hanly and Pierratos showed a significant reduction of the apnea-hypopnea index (AHI, normal <5) in all patients after conversion from CHD to nocturnal HHD (AHI from 46 ± 25 to 8 ± 8 per hour; $P < 0.05$).[37] While several other studies support these findings, the effects of more frequent HHD seen on daytime sleepiness and restless legs syndrome have not been as significant. However, observational studies have shown improvement of restless leg syndrome after kidney transplantation, most likely attributable to better clearance and volume control, which may be achievable with more frequent HHD.

In summary, daytime sleepiness and sleep disorders are common in patients with ESKD. OSA has been consistently shown to improve after conversion to NHD (five times a week, 6 to 8 hours per session) which warrants wider therapeutic implementation in patients with ESKD.

[For more information, see Chapter 7.]

PREGNANCY AND INTENSIVE HEMODIALYSIS

The first successful pregnancy on dialysis was reported in 1970. However, pregnancies in patients with ESKD continue to be rare, with pregnancies beyond the third trimester as low as 0.3 per 100 patient-years.[38] With the introduction of erythropoietin as a therapeutic agent, increasing HD dose, and advances in HD membrane technology, pregnancies have become more frequent. However, the likelihood of successful pregnancies in women with ESKD undergoing CHD is still significantly lower than in the general population. In fact, one study reported that 1.1% versus 2.4% of women of childbearing age on PD versus CHD, respectively, became pregnant over a 4-year period.[39]

In general, fertility along with maternal and fetal well-being are prerequisites for a successful and uncomplicated pregnancy, all of which are affected by ESKD. Fertility is markedly decreased due to low levels of progesterone and estrogen and most patients experience amenorrhea.[40] Even among women with regular menses, most have anovulatory cycles. Increased maternal risks of pregnancy in ESKD include gestational HTN, preeclampsia, and HELLP (hemolysis, elevated liver enzymes, low platelets). Additionally, greater need for blood transfusions had been noted, with associated increased likelihood of sensitization complicating future kidney transplantation. Finally, fetal risks, including intrauterine growth restriction, spontaneous abortion, and premature labor, are common.

Better clearance and volume control via intensive HD increase the chances of a successful pregnancy. After switching to intensive HD, regular menses often recur after 3 months.[40] While there are no definitive studies showing a direct link between changes in biochemical parameters and the rate of conception, a study from Toronto showed an increased rate of pregnancies in a cohort of 45 women undergoing intensive HD.[41,42]

Pregnancies occur more frequently on intensive HD and have better maternal and fetal outcomes. The most comprehensive data come from a Canadian retrospective study comparing a cohort of 17 patients with 22 pregnancies to 70 pregnancies from the American Pregnancy Registry Cohort.[41] There was a direct relationship between the hours of HD per week and live birth rate, with a 48% live birth rate among women dialyzing 20 hours or less a week compared to up to 85% in women dialyzing 36 hours or more per week. Furthermore, gestational age in the intensively dialyzed group was significantly higher (median 36 weeks vs. 27 weeks). Additionally, pregnant patients undergoing NHD had better blood pressure control with lower incidence of preeclampsia and a higher incidence of vaginal delivery.[41]

While the dose of HD plays a pivotal role in improving fertility and pregnancy outcomes, the care for women with ESKD who seek to become pregnant include all aspects of pregnancy care, from preconception counseling to postpartum care. Since the maternal and fetal risks remain elevated in patients with ESKD, contraception is important for all women who do not wish to get pregnant. Once a woman decides she wants to become pregnant, she should be informed about the risks of pregnancies in ESKD and the potential benefits of an intensified HD schedule. It is important to note that pregnancy in the setting of ESKD must have close maternal and fetal monitoring by a combined obstetrical and nephrology team. In the first trimester, monthly appointments are usually sufficient, but should increase to weekly appointments in the last trimester.

Follow-up care includes standard care such as screening for fetal abnormalities and evaluating for maternal complications like preeclampsia, HELLP, gestational diabetes, and anemia. HD-specific considerations include increased need for erythropoiesis-stimulating agents (ESAs) and water-soluble vitamins, and titration of target weight. Due to an increased risk for preeclampsia, aspirin use may be advised in the absence of contraindications. Given the increased risk of cervical incompetence, cervical length is monitored every 2 weeks after week 20. Vaginal delivery is safe in most patients. Induction at 37 weeks is recommended due to the lack of benefits of gestational age beyond this point. If magnesium is used in the pre- or peri-delivery period, dose reduction may be necessary in anuric patients due to increased risk of accumulation and toxicity.[43]

Most aspects of postpartum care in patients with ESKD are similar to the general population. A new baby is challenging for all parents and may pose as an additional burden for patients doing intensive HD at home. In-center dialysis may be offered and discussed with patients for the immediate post-partum period.

[For more information, see Chapter 7.]

▌ HOME HEMODIALYSIS IN CHILDREN

Treatment of ESKD in children poses a different challenge. Like adults, children with ESKD must manage HTN and minimize risks of developing vascular calcification. However, there are several complications that are unique to children. Body growth and, even more importantly, brain development make children especially vulnerable to metabolic disturbances. In fact, a systematic review showed that CKD in children is associated with poorer neurocognitive performance compared to their peers and the burden of uremic toxins is believed to play a pivotal role in the pathogenesis of these findings.[44]

Children receive priority for deceased-donor kidney transplantation and therefore wait times are usually significantly shorter than in adults. However, patients without a living donor usually cannot undergo preemptive transplantation and need dialysis for a period of time. Vascular access can be challenging in children. Therefore, PD is the modality of choice, particularly in children under the age of 5. There are no randomized studies investigating the effects of intensifying dialysis in children—only small case series (12 patients in the largest series) are available. These studies have shown benefits such as better blood pressure and volume control, improved calcium-phosphate metabolism, liberation of diet and volume intake, and a lesser pill burden.[45] Data on specific pediatrics outcomes such as better school attendance and growth are scarce and inconsistent. However, some reports suggest improved growth without the need of growth hormone supplementation.[46]

While there is no definite minimum age for HHD, certain centers use a cutoff of 20 kg or more as an inclusion criterion. For children younger than 16 years, ideally two adults are trained in HHD for an average duration of 6 to 8 weeks. It is important that parents understand the responsibilities and amount of work required for HHD in children. Prescribing HHD in children depends mainly on weight and is prescribed on an individual basis. SDHD as well as NHD prescriptions are possible and depend on physicians' and patients' preference. In the United States, mostly low dialysate flow machines are used with the advantage of compact size and transportability. Once at home, pediatric patients need close follow-up every 4 to 8 weeks depending on medical stability. As for home dialysis in general, around-the-clock support and a clear plan for emergency situations are crucial.

▍REFRACTORY ASCITES

Refractory ascites in patients with ESKD is a particular challenge to nephrologists due to intradialytic hemodynamic instability. Cirrhosis, cancer, and HF are the most common conditions associated with ascites, accounting for 81%, 10%, and 3% of patients, respectively. Portal HTN induces production of vasodilators and splanchnic vasodilatation with reduced total peripheral resistance. Hypotension tends to prohibit adequate volume control, especially during short dialysis sessions. PD has been shown to be feasible in patients with ascites with the advantage of gentler UF. Additionally, PD offers regular removal of ascites without the need for repeat paracentesis. However, PD also has limitations that include excessive albumin loss, peritonitis, and malnutrition.

Increasing HD time, usually to more than 30 hours per week, offers excellent volume control not only through shorter interval between sessions with lesser fluid accumulation, but also slower UF over a longer time period mitigating intradialytic hypotension (IDH). Use of more frequent HHD in refractory ascites is limited to case reports, but excellent ascites control has been reported. In a patient with ascites presumably due to membranous nephropathy with nephrotic syndrome, ascites resolved completely after 12 weeks of HHD with 8-hour treatments 6 days a week. Interestingly, ascites immediately reoccurred after only 2 weeks undergoing CHD while on vacation and resolved again after resuming more frequent HHD. IDH and cramping being regularly occurring on CHD was well controlled after conversion to more frequent HHD.[47] In another patient with focal biliary cirrhosis and ascites with ESKD due to calcineurin toxicity, IDH was frequent and ascites did not improve. After initiation of more frequent HHD, ascites resolved completely.[47]

Possible mechanisms to explain improvement in ascites have been suggested. Better volume control due to more frequent and longer HD sessions without hemodynamic compromise leads to reduction in ascites. Furthermore, uremic toxins may reduce peritoneal lymphatic flow and increase peritoneal permeability. Better clearance with intense HD could thereby improve peritoneal functionality and prevent ascites formation. It is also reasonable to hypothesize that improvement in right ventricular function with reduction of venous congestion may lead to correction of ascites.

HOME HEMODIALYSIS AFTER PD TECHNIQUE FAILURE (HOME-TO-HOME TRANSITION)

PD accounts for a much larger proportion of home dialysis patients than does HHD. PD is easier to learn, with most patients needing a few days compared to several weeks of training for HHD. In general, more patients are considered suitable candidates for PD, particularly among older patients who may have multiple comorbidities or disabilities.[48] Patients may perceive that PD allows more flexibility with travel and greater independence (as no care partner is required).

Questions have been raised in regard to possible competition between PD and HHD programs for patients initiating home dialysis; however, these modalities seem more to complement each other.[49,50] Despite the above-mentioned differences, PD and HHD share important commonalities. Both PD and HHD patients value independence. Additionally, former PD patients already have experience in self-care. A significant proportion of patients on PD experience technique failure long before nearing the end of life. Those not suitable or waiting for kidney transplantation constitute a distinctive group suited for HHD. Identifying these patients to offer HHD is crucial and several studies have reported on predictors of patients switching to HHD after PD.[51]

HHD as a salvage therapy for PD patients has been shown to be feasible, with most patients having improved clearance on HHD. Cumulative technique and patient survival on HHD did not show any difference between former PD and PD naïve patients.[52] However, time to hospitalization was shorter in patients with previous PD exposure. In another study, survival was better on HHD compared to CHD. Overall, patients with previous PD exposure initiating HHD after technique failure are younger and, while having more comorbidities than patients without former PD exposure, are still healthier than the general PD population.[53]

Taken together, HHD seems to be an obvious choice for many patients after PD failure, giving them the opportunity to stay independent and benefit from the additional biochemical and clinical advantages of increased clearance. However, only a small fraction of such patients actually pursue HHD. One reason for this may be the above-mentioned increased morbidity in PD patients, especially after years on renal replacement therapy (RRT). Additionally, "traditional" patient barriers to HHD such as fear of self-needling, complexity of treatment with perceived burden on family members, and fear of catastrophic events may play a pivotal role.[54] Finally, lack of HHD experience and training among treating nephrologists and the lack of an established HHD program could further prevent PD patients from switching to HHD.

In summary, HHD is a feasible and an attractive option for patients with PD technique failure who do not qualify for, or are awaiting, kidney transplantation. However, few patients actually pursue HHD after PD and further strategies to facilitate home-to-home transition are needed.[55]

▌ HOME HEMODIALYSIS IN ELDERLY PATIENTS

In a survey published in 1984, almost half of all nephrologists who were asked whether they would offer RRT to a 50-year-old patient with ischemic heart disease answered "no."[56] While reasons for rejection were not reported in this study, age and multisystem disease were the strongest predictors of rejection. Over 30 years later, according to the USRDS, 23% of patients who initiated RRT in 2015 were 75 years or older. The vast majority started HD (94%), while the remainder pursued PD (5.9%) or kidney transplant (0.1%). Older patients appear more likely to do CHD when they reach ESKD. Many have worsening of functional status after dialysis initiation, requiring increased support from care partners or transfer to nursing homes. The initiation of a life-changing therapy and its complications contribute to this decline. Most elderly patients are vulnerable due to "geriatric syndromes" consisting of frailty, disabilities, delirium, falls, cognitive impairment, and incontinence. To understand the possible benefits of HHD in the elderly, it is important to identify problems and pitfalls of CHD in this population.

Hypotension during HD is associated with increased morbidity and mortality. Elderly patients are particularly prone to blood pressure variations during HD. Impaired cardiac function (systolic and diastolic), arterial stiffness, and reduced oncotic pressure leading to delayed vascular refilling along with reduced autonomic nervous system reactivity contribute to IDH. As a consequence, significant hypoperfusion of major organs occurs. Myocardial stunning is one of the best described effects, with fibrotic changes and cardiac dysfunction over time further promoting hypotensive episodes. Other organs affected by (repeated) insults are the brain and the gut. Interestingly, subcortical ischemia has been shown to be associated with mood disorders often occurring soon after dialysis initiation.[57] Other subcortical functions include decision making and executive functions, both often already diminished in elderly patients, further increasing the chances of losing independence. Ischemia of the gut can lead to barrier dysfunction with translocation of proinflammatory endotoxins resulting in inflammation, wasting, and malnutrition. Inadequate dialysis, polypharmacy, poor dental status, and constipation can contribute to poor nutritional status. Intercurrent illnesses also play an important role. Finally, decreased immunological response of leukocytes in the uremic milieu to pathogens increases susceptibility to infections. Decreased response to vaccines further complicates the immunologic status, with infections being a main cause of mortality in the elderly.[58]

More frequent HHD has the potential to address several of these challenges. As discussed previously, hypotensive episodes occur less frequently with more frequent HHD. Blood pressure control and LVH improve with HHD. A study by Jassal et al. also found signs of cerebral protection with better cognitive function in patients converting from CHD to HHD.[59] Liberalization of diet on HHD along with better clearance of uremic toxins lead to better appetite and increased muscle mass as signs of improved nutrition status. Better clearance may also lead to improved immune status and lesser infections.

Despite these potential benefits in elderly patients, several challenges remain. Self-care is often not feasible and more frequent HHD at home may become overwhelming to the patient. Even if a care partner is willing to help, a significant commitment is needed. Rehabilitation programs with integrated dialysis can help patients to successfully complete HHD training, but such programs are not widely established.[60] PD in the nursing home is relatively well established; while HHD in nursing homes is feasible, it is significantly more labor intensive and demanding to nursing home staff. Despite these challenges, HHD has not only been shown to be possible in older people, but has also resulted in high patient satisfaction.[61] To successfully initiate HHD in elderly patients, a multidisciplinary approach with physicians, nurses, social workers, dieticians along with family members is crucial. Overall, giving patients the options to choose between dialysis modalities can improve quality of life. Home modalities should not be withheld from the growing geriatric patient population.[58]

▌REFERENCES

1. Tennankore K, Nadeau-Fredette AC, Chan CT. Intensified home hemodialysis: clinical benefits, risks and target populations. *Nephrol Dial Transplant.* 2014;29:1342-1349.
2. Collins AJ, Foley RN, Gilbertson DT, Chen SC. The state of chronic kidney disease, ESRD, and morbidity and mortality in the first year of dialysis. *Clin J Am Soc Nephrol.* 2009;4(suppl 1):S5-S11.
3. Chan CT. Cardiovascular effects of home intensive hemodialysis. *Adv Chronic Kidney Dis.* 2009;16:173-178.
4. Chan CT, Floras JS, Miller JA, Richardson RM, Pierratos A. Regression of left ventricular hypertrophy after conversion to nocturnal hemodialysis. *Kidney Int.* 2002;61:2235-2239.
5. Chan CT, Harvey PJ, Picton P, Pierratos A, Miller JA, Floras JS. Short-term blood pressure, noradrenergic, and vascular effects of nocturnal home hemodialysis. *Hypertension.* 2003;42:925-931.
6. McCullough PA, Chan CT, Weinhandl ED, Burkart JM, Bakris GL. Intensive hemodialysis, left ventricular hypertrophy, and cardiovascular disease. *Am J Kidney Dis.* 2016;68:S5-S14.
7. Agarwal R, Nissenson AR, Batlle D, Coyne DW, Trout JR, Warnock DG. Prevalence, treatment, and control of hypertension in chronic hemodialysis patients in the United States. *Am J Med.* 2003;115:291-297.
8. Kjellstrand CM, Evans RL, Petersen RJ, Shideman JR, von Hartitzsch B, Buselmeier TJ. The "unphysiology" of dialysis: a major cause of dialysis side effects? *Kidney Int Suppl.* 1975;(2):30-34.
9. Fagugli RM, Reboldi G, Quintaliani G, et al. Short daily hemodialysis: blood pressure control and left ventricular mass reduction in hypertensive hemodialysis patients. *Am J Kidney Dis.* 2001;38:371-376.
10. Chan CT, Lovren F, Pan Y, Verma S. Nocturnal haemodialysis is associated with improved vascular smooth muscle cell biology. *Nephrol Dial Transplant.* 2009;24:3867-3871.
11. Chan CT, Mardirossian S, Faratro R, Richardson RM. Improvement in lower-extremity peripheral arterial disease by nocturnal hemodialysis. *Am J Kidney Dis.* 2003;41:225-229.
12. Chan CT, Jain V, Picton P, Pierratos A, Floras JS. Nocturnal hemodialysis increases arterial baroreflex sensitivity and compliance and normalizes blood pressure of hypertensive patients with end-stage renal disease. *Kidney Int.* 2005;68:338-344.
13. Foley RN. Clinical epidemiology of cardiac disease in dialysis patients: left ventricular hypertrophy, ischemic heart disease, and cardiac failure. *Semin Dial.* 2003;16:111-117.

14. Foley RN. Cardiac disease in chronic uremia: can it explain the reverse epidemiology of hypertension and survival in dialysis patients? *Semin Dial.* 2004;17:275-278.

15. Foley RN, Curtis BM, Randell EW, Parfrey PS. Left ventricular hypertrophy in new hemodialysis patients without symptomatic cardiac disease. *Clin J Am Soc Nephrol.* 2010;5:805-813.

16. Susantitaphong P, Koulouridis I, Balk EM, Madjas NE, Jaber BL. Effect of frequent or extended hemodialysis on cardiovascular parameters: a meta-analysis. *Am J Kidney Dis.* 2012;59(5):689-699.

17. Chan CT, Greene T, Chertow GM, et al. Determinants of left ventricular mass in patients on hemodialysis: Frequent Hemodialysis Network (FHN) trials. *Circ Cardiovasc Imaging.* 2012;5:251-261.

18. Trinh E, Chan CT. Intensive home hemodialysis results in regression of left ventricular hypertrophy and better clinical outcomes. *Am J Nephrol.* 2016;44:300-307.

19. Chan C, Floras JS, Miller JA, Pierratos A. Improvement in ejection fraction by nocturnal haemodialysis in end-stage renal failure patients with coexisting heart failure. *Nephrol Dial Transplant.* 2002;17:1518-1521.

20. Fabbian F, Cantelli S, Molino C, Pala M, Longhini C, Portaluppi F. Pulmonary hypertension in dialysis patients: a cross-sectional Italian study. *Int J Nephrol.* 2010;2011:283475.

21. Raimann JG, Chan CT, Daugirdas JT, et al. The effect of increased frequency of hemodialysis on volume-related outcomes: a secondary analysis of the frequent hemodialysis network trials. *Blood Purif.* 2016;41:277-286.

22. Chan CT, Greene T, Chertow GM, et al. Effects of frequent hemodialysis on ventricular volumes and left ventricular remodeling. *Clin J Am Soc Nephrol.* 2013;8:2106-2116.

23. Girsberger M, Thenganatt J, Chan CT. Correction of pulmonary hypertension with intensive hemodialysis: a case report. *Hemodial Int.* 2019;23:E49-E52.

24. Ketteler M, Biggar PH, Liangos O. FGF23 antagonism: the thin line between adaptation and maladaptation in chronic kidney disease. *Nephrol Dial Transplant.* 2013;28:821-825.

25. Chan CT. Nocturnal hemodialysis: an attempt to correct the "unphysiology" of conventional intermittent renal replacement therapy. *Clin Invest Med.* 2002;25:233-235.

26. Rocco MV, Lockridge RS Jr, Beck GJ, et al. The effects of frequent nocturnal home hemodialysis: the Frequent Hemodialysis Network Nocturnal Trial. *Kidney Int.* 2011;80:1080-1091.

27. Ayus JC, Achinger SG, Mizani MR, et al. Phosphorus balance and mineral metabolism with 3 h daily hemodialysis. *Kidney Int.* 2007;71:336-342.

28. Mucsi I, Hercz G, Uldall R, Ouwendyk M, Francoeur R, Pierratos A. Control of serum phosphate without any phosphate binders in patients treated with nocturnal hemodialysis. *Kidney Int.* 1998;53:1399-1404.

29. Ayus JC, Mizani MR, Achinger SG, Thadhani R, Go AS, Lee S. Effects of short daily versus conventional hemodialysis on left ventricular hypertrophy and inflammatory markers: a prospective, controlled study. *J Am Soc Nephrol.* 2005;16:2778-2788.

30. Perl J, Unruh ML, Chan CT. Sleep disorders in end-stage renal disease: 'markers of inadequate dialysis'? *Kidney Int.* 2006;70:1687-1693.
31. Elias RM, Bradley TD, Kasai T, Motwani SS, Chan CT. Rostral overnight fluid shift in end-stage renal disease: relationship with obstructive sleep apnea. *Nephrol Dial Transplant.* 2012;27:1569-1573.
32. Elias RM, Chan CT, Paul N, et al. Relationship of pharyngeal water content and jugular volume with severity of obstructive sleep apnea in renal failure. *Nephrol Dial Transplant.* 2013;28:937-944.
33. Parker KP. Sleep disturbances in dialysis patients. *Sleep Med Rev.* 2003;7:131-143.
34. Furst P. Amino acid metabolism in uremia. *J Am Coll Nutr.* 1989;8:310-323.
35. Soreide E, Skeie B, Kirvela O, et al. Branched-chain amino acid in chronic renal failure patients: respiratory and sleep effects. *Kidney Int.* 1991;40:539-543.
36. Tang SC, Lam B, Lai AS, et al. Improvement in sleep apnea during nocturnal peritoneal dialysis is associated with reduced airway congestion and better uremic clearance. *Clin J Am Soc Nephrol.* 2009;4:410-418.
37. Hanly PJ, Pierratos A. Improvement of sleep apnea in patients with chronic renal failure who undergo nocturnal hemodialysis. *N Engl J Med.* 2001;344:102-107.
38. Bagon JA, Vernaeve H, De Muylder X, Lafontaine JJ, Martens J, Van Roost G. Pregnancy and dialysis. *Am J Kidney Dis.* 1998;31:756-765.
39. Okundaye I, Abrinko P, Hou S. Registry of pregnancy in dialysis patients. *Am J Kidney Dis.* 1998;31:766-773.
40. van Eps C, Hawley C, Jeffries J, et al. Changes in serum prolactin, sex hormones and thyroid function with alternate nightly nocturnal home haemodialysis. *Nephrology (Carlton).* 2012;17:42-47.
41. Hladunewich MA, Hou S, Odutayo A, et al. Intensive hemodialysis associates with improved pregnancy outcomes: a Canadian and United States cohort comparison. *J Am Soc Nephrol.* 2014;25:1103-1109.
42. Barua M, Hladunewich M, Keunen J, et al. Successful pregnancies on nocturnal home hemodialysis. *Clin J Am Soc Nephrol.* 2008;3:392-396.
43. Hladunewich M, Hercz AE, Keunen J, Chan C, Pierratos A. Pregnancy in end stage renal disease. *Semin Dial.* 2011;24:634-639.
44. Ruebner RL, Laney N, Kim JY, et al. Neurocognitive dysfunction in children, adolescents, and young adults with CKD. *Am J Kidney Dis.* 2016;67:567-575.
45. Geary DF, Piva E, Tyrrell J, et al. Home nocturnal hemodialysis in children. *J Pediatr.* 2005;147:383-387.
46. Hothi DK, Stronach L, Sinnott K. Home hemodialysis in children. *Hemodial Int.* 2016;20:349-57.
47. Pauly RP, Sood MM, Chan CT. Management of refractory ascites using nocturnal home hemodialysis. *Semin Dial.* 2008;21:367-370.
48. Rioux JP, Bargman JM, Chan CT. Systematic differences among patients initiated on home haemodialysis and peritoneal dialysis: the fallacy of potential competition. *Nephrol Dial Transplant.* 2010;25:2364-2367.
49. Shah N, Quinn RR, Thompson S, Pauly RP. Can home hemodialysis and peritoneal dialysis programs coexist and grow together? *Perit Dial Int.* 2017;37:591-594.

50. Nadeau-Fredette AC, Hawley CM, Pascoe EM, et al. An incident cohort study comparing survival on home hemodialysis and peritoneal dialysis (Australia and New Zealand Dialysis and Transplantation Registry). *Clin J Am Soc Nephrol.* 2015;10:1397-1407.

51. Nadeau-Fredette AC, Hawley C, Pascoe E, et al. Predictors of transfer to home hemodialysis after peritoneal dialysis completion. *Perit Dial Int.* 2016;36:547-554.

52. Nadeau-Fredette AC, Bargman JM, Chan CT. Clinical outcome of home hemodialysis in patients with previous peritoneal dialysis exposure: evaluation of the integrated home dialysis model. *Perit Dial Int.* 2015;35:316-323.

53. Kansal SK, Morfin JA, Weinhandl ED. Survival and kidney transplant incidence on home versus in-center hemodialysis, following peritoneal dialysis technique failure. *Perit Dial Int.* 2019;39:25-34.

54. Cafazzo JA, Leonard K, Easty AC, Rossos PG, Chan CT. Patient-perceived barriers to the adoption of nocturnal home hemodialysis. *Clin J Am Soc Nephrol.* 2009;4:784-789.

55. McCormick BB, Chan CT, ORN Home Dialysis Research Group. Striving to achieve an integrated home dialysis system: a report from the Ontario Renal Network Home Dialysis Attrition Task Force. *Clin J Am Soc Nephrol.* 2018;13:468-470.

56. Challah S, Wing AJ, Bauer R, Morris RW, Schroeder SA. Negative selection of patients for dialysis and transplantation in the United Kingdom. *Br Med J (Clin Res Ed).* 1984;288:1119-1122.

57. Lamar M, Charlton RA, Morris RG, Markus HS. The impact of subcortical white matter disease on mood in euthymic older adults: a diffusion tensor imaging study. *Am J Geriatr Psychiatry.* 2010;18:634-642.

58. Auguste BL, Chan CT. Home dialysis among elderly patients: outcomes and future directions. *Can J Kidney Health Dis.* 2019;6:2054358119871031.

59. Jassal SV, Devins GM, Chan CT, Bozanovic R, Rourke S. Improvements in cognition in patients converting from thrice weekly hemodialysis to nocturnal hemodialysis: a longitudinal pilot study. *Kidney Int.* 2006;70:956-962.

60. Ibrahim A, Chan CT. Managing kidney failure with home hemodialysis. *Clin J Am Soc Nephrol.* 2019;14:1268-1273.

61. Derrett S, Darmody M, Williams S, Rutherford M, Schollum J, Walker R. Older peoples' satisfaction with home-based dialysis. *Nephrology (Carlton).* 2010;15:464-470.

POLICY AND COSTS OF HOME HEMODIALYSIS

14

Michael A. Kraus and Eric Weinhandl

Home hemodialysis (HHD) is the least utilized dialytic modality in the United States, behind both in-center hemodialysis (HD) and peritoneal dialysis (PD). Nevertheless, since the end of 2002, when there were only 1519 HHD patients in the United States, the size of the HHD patient population has more than quintupled.[1] Policy considerations have played an important role in the expansion of HHD, with some policies encouraging growth and other policies discouraging growth.

∎ PRACTICE POLICY

Much of the delivery of HHD is governed by the Medicare Survey and Certification Program, which specifies safety and quality standards, otherwise known as Conditions for Coverage (CfC). Regarding dialysis in the home setting, these standards address the requirements of HHD training, the frequency of HHD patient monitoring, and the breadth of support services, including home visits and water quality assessments. These standards were revised in 2008. At the same time, the Centers for Medicare & Medicaid Services (CMS) also issued interpretive guidance that describes for state surveyors the implications of each standard. Because the standards do require interpretation, states may ultimately permit or deny specific provider practices pertaining to HHD delivery.

In addition to regulation by CMS and state departments of health, the US Food and Drug Administration (FDA) must evaluate HHD equipment and supplies. In practice, dialysis machines are evaluated initially in the facility setting, with emphasis on successful completion of treatments and delivery of minimally adequate small-solute clearance (e.g., as quantified by single-pool or standardized Kt/V). After a machine is cleared for use in the facility setting, the manufacturer may initiate an investigational device exemption (IDE) trial—typically employing a crossover design—that evaluates whether the machine delivers either equivalent or non-inferior treatment in the home setting. The evaluation of an IDE trial forms the basis of FDA clearance for use in the home setting. This clearance includes specific product-labeling instructions that may create limitations on use of the machine in the home setting. For this reason, additional trials may be necessary to evaluate whether a machine is cleared for nocturnal HHD or HHD without a care partner, as examples. Without additional clearances, specific applications of the machine are considered "off label," thus creating potential liabilities that may lead healthcare providers to draft internal policies that prohibit or discourage those applications.

❚ PAYMENT POLICY

Arguably, the most important part of policy concerning HHD is payment. Because most dialysis patients carry either Medicare Parts A and B (i.e., fee-for-service) coverage or Medicare Part C (i.e., Medicare Advantage) coverage, the payment policies promulgated by CMS can have a tremendous impact on the economics of HHD.

For all patients newly diagnosed with end-stage kidney disease (ESKD), CMS requires submission of form CMS-2728, the "End Stage Renal Disease Medical Evidence Report: Medicare Entitlement and/or Patient Registration." Usually, Medicare entitlement begins on the first day of the third calendar month after the calendar month in which the patient begins chronic dialysis. This 3-month "qualifying period" may be waived if a patient begins a self-care dialysis training program in a Medicare-approved training facility and is expected to self-dialyze after the completion of the training program. Therefore, this waiver applies to both PD and HHD. PD is typically prescribed as an initial dialytic therapy, while HHD is often prescribed later in the course of ESKD. Weinhandl et al. reported that in a cohort of 4201 HHD patients using NxStage equipment, mean ESKD duration prior to HHD initiation was approximately 45 months.[2] This is not unique to the United States. Merely 0.4% of incident dialysis patients in the United States were prescribed

HHD in 2017. Similarly, only 0.7% of incident dialysis patients in Canada were prescribed HHD in 2018.[1,3] In any case, if an incident dialysis patient were to begin HHD training, that patient would be eligible for Medicare coverage from the first day of ESKD. This may be an overlooked matter in patients without preexisting Medicare coverage.

Since the advent of the Prospective Payment System in 2011, reimbursement for each outpatient dialysis treatment during the first 120 Medicare-eligible days after initiation of chronic dialysis has been inflated by the "onset of dialysis" adjustment. At present, the multiplier of the base payment rate is equal to 1.33. Thus, while an outpatient HD treatment covered by Medicare Part B carries an allowable charge of approximately $240 in the long run, each treatment during the first 120 days carries an allowable charge of approximately $320. This may also be relevant to the provision of HHD, as the cost of training a patient is formidable.

For HHD training, Medicare extends an add-on payment for each training session that occurs after the first 120 days following initiation of chronic dialysis. For PD, up to 15 training sessions may be covered. However, for HHD, up to 25 training sessions may be covered. Each add-on payment is currently equal to nearly $50. Because the majority of new HHD patients are prevalent dialysis patients, this training add-on payment is typically available.

Although initial Medicare eligibility and payment for HHD training are both important considerations in the short run, the long-term economics of HHD are dictated by two significant issues, payment for additional HD sessions and the monthly capitated payment (MCP) to the nephrologist who supervises the care of the HHD patient.

With respect to additional HD sessions, Medicare has long declared that it will reimburse dialysis providers for a maximum of 13 outpatient HD treatments in a 30-day month or 14 outpatient HD treatments in a 31-day month. This reimbursement is justified by the diagnosis of ESKD itself; for that reason, a claim requires only the International Classification of Diseases, 10th Edition, Clinical Modification (ICD-10-CM) diagnosis code N18.6, "end-stage renal disease." Any patient may dialyze more frequently than 13 times in a 30-day month or 14 times in a 31-day month, but the dialysis provider will not be reimbursed for so-called additional HD sessions unless they are medically justified. This is an important issue unique to the United States. Currently, the vast majority of HHD patients in the United States use equipment that utilizes a low volume of dialysate. Many patients dialyze during daytime hours, with session duration of 2 to 3 hours and dialysate volume of 20 to 40 L. To achieve guideline-recommended HD adequacy in this specific framework, as indicated by a minimum standardized Kt/V equal to 2.1 and a target standardized Kt/V

equal to 2.3, HD frequency between four and six sessions per week is often necessary; for small patients (i.e., with low total body water volume), for patients with clinically significant residual renal function, and for patients who are dialyzing nocturnally, three sessions may be minimally adequate. Therefore, in the United States, but not in other high-income countries, HHD and frequent HD are practically synonymous.

CMS does not have a national coverage decision regarding HD frequency. Instead, policy about payment for additional HD sessions is dictated by the local coverage determinations of the Medicare administrative contractors (MACs). In 2019, the MACs harmonized their individual policies about payment for additional HD sessions. In general, payment for additional HD sessions will be rendered if those sessions are determined to be "reasonable and necessary" for the treatment of specific medical conditions. The broad categories of conditions comprise metabolic conditions (acidosis, hyperkalemia, and hyperphosphatemia); fluid-positive status not otherwise controlled with routine, thrice-weekly HD; pregnancy; heart failure; pericarditis; and incomplete dialysis secondary to either hypotension or vascular access complications. Medicare claims that seek reimbursement must include one or more specific ICD-10-CM diagnosis codes pertaining to those conditions; the local coverage determinations include billing articles that specify which diagnosis codes may be used. In all cases, the plan of care must include detailed, supportive documentation. Commercial insurers publish qualitatively similar policies regarding payment.

The MCP is another important consideration. In each calendar month, a physician may submit a Medicare Part B claim for dialysis-related physician services that are furnished to a chronic dialysis patient. For adult patients, there are four current procedural terminology (CPT) codes that may be used when a physician furnishes a full month of care: 90960, for in-center HD patients who are seen four or more times; 90961, for in-center HD patients who are seen two or three times; 90962, for in-center HD patients who are seen one time; and 90966, for home dialysis patients, regardless of dialytic modality and visit frequency. Reimbursement rates for each of these codes are determined by relative value units (RVUs). Current, the numbers of RVUs assigned to 90961 and 90966 are equal. In other words, a physician currently receives equal payments for the care of in-center HD patients who are seen (usually in the dialysis facility) two or three times in a month and for the care of home dialysis patients. However, the number of RVUs assigned to 90960 is higher. Thus, in practice, a physician who sees an in-center HD patient once per week in the dialysis facility will receive a larger MCP than a physician who sees an HHD patient once per month in the home dialysis clinic. Whether this encourages or discourages the prescription of HHD is unclear.[4] Nevertheless, CMS recognizes that this disparity exists and has declared during annual rulemaking that the CPT codes for the MCP are potentially misvalued. However, no action has yet been taken to revise the physician fee schedule. Voluntary payment models that have been recently proposed by the Centers for Medicare and Medicaid Innovation (CMMI) endeavor to eliminate this disparity.

■ ECONOMICS OF HOME HEMODIALYSIS

There are no national studies of the economics of HHD in the United States. The United States Renal Data System (USRDS) reports economic analyses about HD, regardless of setting, and PD. At present, per person per year (PPPY) Medicare expenditures on HHD are unknown. However, because analyses of Medicare claims have suggested that the all-cause hospital admission rates with frequent HHD and thrice-weekly in-center HD are nearly equal (given appropriate risk adjustment), it is likely that PPPY Medicare expenditures on HHD patients are roughly equal to corresponding expenditures on in-center HD patients. In other high-income countries, including Australia and Canada, HHD is associated with lower costs than in-center HD.[5] However, frequency of HD has a significant impact. Conventional HHD is less costly than intensive HHD in many analyses. However, choice of equipment also matters. In a recent study of dialysis economics in the Canadian province of Manitoba, training costs with conventional equipment were substantially higher than training costs with NxStage equipment.[6]

Aside from costs to payers, the cost of HHD to patients and their families must also be considered. Electricity and water expenditures with HHD are likely to increase, especially when equipment consumes a high volume of dialysate per treatment. These costs may not be waived by local governments and utilities, although medical hardship programs do exist. Some patients may require home renovations to facilitate HHD. In the Frequent Hemodialysis Network (FHN) trial of nocturnal HHD, the median home renovation cost was roughly $1200 in Virginia and $4000 in the Canadian province of Ontario.[7]

Ultimately, the relative economics of HHD versus in-center HD in the United States will primarily depend, for the foreseeable future, on the balance between the cost of additional HD sessions and savings associated with fewer hospitalizations, due to improved volume management and cardiovascular health. At present, additional HD sessions typically create expense for payers. However, if intensive HHD lowers the risk of cardiovascular hospitalization and does not increase the risk of infection-related hospitalization, then the relative economics of HHD versus in-center HD will likely be neutral, if not favorable.

▌REFERENCES

1. Saran R, Robinson B, Abbott KC, et al. US Renal Data System 2019 Annual Data Report: epidemiology of kidney disease in the United States. *Am J Kidney Dis.* 2020;75(1 suppl 1):A6-A7.
2. Weinhandl ED, Gilbertson DT, Collins AJ. Mortality, hospitalization, and technique failure in daily home hemodialysis and matched peritoneal dialysis patients: a matched cohort study. *Am J Kidney Dis.* 2016;67(1):98-110.
3. Canadian Institute for Health Information. Treatment of end-stage organ failure in Canada, Canadian Organ Replacement Register, 2009 to 2018: end-stage kidney disease and kidney transplants—data tables; 2019.
4. Manns B, Agar JWM, Biyani M, et al. Can economic incentives increase the use of home dialysis? *Nephrol Dial Transplant.* 2019;34(5):731-741.
5. Walker RC, Howard K, Morton RL. Home hemodialysis: a comprehensive review of patient-centered and economic considerations. *Clin Outcomes Res.* 2017;9:149-161.
6. Beaudry A, Ferguson TW, Rigatto C, Tangri N, Dumanski S, Komenda P. Cost of dialysis therapy by modality in Manitoba. *Clin J Am Soc Nephrol.* 2018;13(8):1197-1203.
7. Pipkin M, Eggers PW, Larive B, et al. Recruitment and training for home hemodialysis: experience and lessons from the Nocturnal Dialysis Trial. *Clin J Am Soc Nephrol.* 2010;5(9):1614-1620.

SETTING UP, BUILDING, AND SUSTAINING A HOME DIALYSIS PROGRAM

15

Nupur Gupta and Brent W. Miller

Outpatient home hemodialysis (HHD) began contemporaneously in the 1960s with chronic center-based hemodialysis (HD) and before the routine provision of home peritoneal dialysis (PD).[1] Prior to the establishment of the Medicare End-Stage Renal Disease program in 1973 in the United States, approximately 40% of US dialysis patients were treated with HHD, although the patient demographics and clinical conditions were much different than today.[2] Over the following decade, home-based PD and conventional thrice-weekly facility-based HD—with over 7000 locations currently—overwhelmed HHD. The subsequent elimination of any assistance on care partner financial support and the economic unfeasibility of staff-assisted HHD further pushed HHD to near extinction by the late 1990s. As a result, a substantial number of nephrologists have neither encountered an HHD patient nor observed a treatment.[3,4]

From this nadir, the prevalence of HHD has nearly tripled over the last 15 years for a variety of reasons, and this trend is expected to continue.[2,3,5] In order to provide adequate access to HHD, more HHD programs will be needed with engaged nephrologists participating in the program-building process. This chapter will focus on setting up, building, and sustaining an HHD program, mainly based on practices in North America. A well-developed strategic plan that addresses financial sustainability, practical logistical issues, and administrative policies are the foundation of a successful program.

▌PLANNING

Size

The first step in developing an HHD program is to estimate its ultimate size. Estimation of scale is a relatively straightforward process but is rarely handled well. First, one should determine the potential geographic "catchment area." Then, obtain the number of end-stage kidney disease (ESKD) patients within the geographic area, and after discussion with several nephrologists, determine what percentage of patients are potential home dialysis patients (10% to 40% is the current range). Lastly, ascertain what the most likely breakdown between PD and HHD will be (65%:35% is a reasonable place to start). No further steps should be taken—as the correct course of action depends upon the interpretation of these results—until all stakeholders concur on these issues.

Management and Ownership

The next step is deciding who will have ownership of the dialysis center and who will be responsible for managing the center. This identifies the entity that has control over decision-making and the culture that is fostered in the home dialysis program. Home dialysis programs cannot succeed without appropriate allocation of resources and a supportive culture, which is difficult to change once established. The variety of ownership and management structures available are beyond the scope of this text, but all should be considered.

Administrative Tasks

In the United States, the Centers for Medicare & Medicaid Services (CMS) certifies every new facility that offers any form of dialysis therapy. No payment from CMS for dialysis is made until successful certification. The prolonged wait for certification can be a financial challenge for any new dialysis center. CMS Conditions for Coverage (CfC) require a state-based survey after the initial application submission (form CMS-855A) to the regional Medicare administrative contractor (MAC). Additionally, in some states, a Certificate of Need (CON) is mandatory for approval of a new dialysis unit. Redesigning space within an existing center requires recertification as well; this includes adding new training facilities or treatment areas. An agreement with the MAC provisionally allows the facility to bill CMS, but future reimbursement is dependent on completing a state survey and maintaining CfC.

In compliance with CfC, all dialysis facilities require a functioning governing body, which can be one or more persons with direct responsibility for the operation of the dialysis center. The major roles of the governing body are described in Table 15-1.[5] The rationale for this requirement is to maintain local responsibility and accountability for the operation of the facility and to have in-person, clinically engaged, competent nephrology leadership participation. Regular meetings with an agenda, monitored attendance, and meeting minutes should be recorded and distributed.[5,6]

Each dialysis facility must have only one medical director ("each facility must have exactly one specific individual to be responsible for all matters...").[5] In the case of a combined center-based and home-based facility, typically, the medical director will appoint a subordinate tasked with the home medical director's responsibilities. These duties are particularly crucial for the quality assurance and process improvement (QAPI) requirement as the practical issues and metrics for center-based dialysis and home dialysis differ substantially.

Home Dialysis Modalities

HHD is typically intertwined with PD. This allows sharing of resources between programs and acknowledges that many patients will ultimately

Table 15-1   MAJOR ROLES OF DIALYSIS FACILITY GOVERNING BODY
Designate a chief executive officer or administrator
Provide adequate staffing of the dialysis facility
Make medical staff appointments, including the medical director
Ensure geographic location of services
Design an internal grievance procedure for patients
Arrange emergency coverage
Provide communication with ESKD networks
Disclose ownership of the facility and keep a record of governing body membership

Source: Adapted from 42 CFR § 494.180. Centers for Medicare & Medicaid Services, HHS. https://www.govinfo.gov/content/pkg/CFR-2008-title42-vol4/pdf/CFR-2008-title42-vol4-sec494-180.pdf.

perform both types of dialysis at some point. The types of HHD offered will determine the structure of the program and the resources needed. Traditional HHD, staff-assisted HHD, short daily HHD, nocturnal HD, respite HD, backup HD, and transitional care HD are the options that should be considered.

Physical Space

Home dialysis facilities can exist in a smaller space than a traditional dialysis center for obvious reasons, but the design should include an adequate area for supply storage, staff work areas, phlebotomy, patient training, and monthly clinics. While space requirements may be minimal at first, planning for future expansion is essential. State requirements for home dialysis programs should also be investigated. In our experience, the minimum space needed to service 40 home dialysis patients is approximately 2000 square feet. If a significant amount of patient training is done in the home, this may lessen the space requirement. Telehealth may also obviate some of the physical space requirements.

Facility Location

Patient convenience is the most important consideration when selecting the location of the center. Travel distance and time, accessible patient parking, supply loading, and proximity to other local transportation options should be considered. Home dialysis can be more practical among patients living in rural areas; hence, many of the pioneers of home dialysis are from rural states. Increased utilization of home dialysis occurs in regions that are more rural and with increasing distance to a dialysis center.[7,8] Geographic and socioeconomic circumstances vary across the United States and may dictate some aspects of access to home dialysis care.[9]

Design

Many patients transport themselves for training and routine visits. Therefore, secure parking should be available. At the entry, a covered drop-off zone that has sufficient lighting and is compliant with the American with Disabilities Act should be built. A waiting room separated from the clinical areas is essential. It should provide a welcoming environment to enable social interaction and maintain privacy. The patient care areas should be organized and uncluttered and provide space for the key tasks of home dialysis: monthly bloodwork, patient training, retraining, respite care, backup care, and monthly clinic visits. In our experience, the design of home dialysis centers often fails to take into consideration the logistics of busy monthly clinics and post-training care (e.g., vascular access retraining) which limits the efficiency of the clinic as it grows. Adequate work space for the staff—nephrologist, dietitian, nurses, medical assistants, social worker, and administrative personnel—should be included.

▌ PERSONNEL

Required staff are described in the CfC: medical director, administrator, dialysis nurses, dietitian, and social worker. Most well-functioning home dialysis centers off-load routine clinical tasks such as phlebotomy, sample preparation, vital signs, and related issues to medical assistants or dialysis technicians and administrative functions to secretarial employees.

"Staffing for growth" is essential. A new home dialysis center will be very training-intensive and will require a lower patient-to-nurse ratio, perhaps 10:1. Mature centers with a larger census-to-training ratio and ancillary staff may be able to maintain a 20:1 ratio. Many states currently mandate one full-time nurse for every 20 or 25 PD patients.[10]

Medical Director

The CfC, which went into effect October 2008, made the medical director the ultimate authority responsible for all aspects of quality care delivered in the facility and markedly increased the scope of his/her responsibilities. The medical director leads as the chief executive officer of the unit. Medicare requires him/her to be board certified and have 12 consecutive months of experience or training in ESKD.[5] Both finances and quality of care at the unit are within the realm of the medical director's responsibilities. These responsibilities include:

- Creating, reviewing, and updating facility policies and procedures;
- Ensuring appropriate modality education and selection for all patients; and
- Overseeing policies and procedures for all staff.

The same nephrologists that deliver direct patient care should participate in the governing body to ensure that the facility is running correctly. The medical director is not solely held responsible for every aspect of care provided in the dialysis facility but is recognized in multiple sections of the CfC. The facility is ultimately the entity sanctioned by the CMS if a medical director does not carry out his/her responsibilities, but large dialysis organizations have developed agreements that delineate medical director expectations and consequences for underperformance.

Facility performance as assessed by infection rates (peritonitis rate, bloodstream infection rate), water quality (by the Association for the Advancement of Medical Instrumentation water quality standards for dialysis), access events, patient admissions and discharges, and QAPI is ultimately the responsibility of medical director. The training and credentialing of medical personnel, including physicians and patient care technicians, are also the medical director's responsibility as specified in the CfC. A medical director must have in-depth knowledge of the regulations and the operations of the dialysis facility in order to provide safe, high-quality care to patients. Before signing a medical director agreement, a nephrologist should ensure he/she is provided with adequate resources to achieve these goals.

Nursing

Various models of nurse staffing are utilized in home dialysis programs. Most commonly, nurses are cross-trained in both PD and HHD. However, some programs do have dedicated nurses for PD and for HHD. Further, some programs also divide the nursing staff into training nurses and nurse coordinators that manage the patients that have completed training. Regardless of the staffing model utilized, every program must provide clinical and technical support to PD and HHD patients

24 hours a day. The addition of medical assistants, dialysis technicians, and administrative personnel allows for more efficient use of staff resources as the program grows.

Social Worker

The nephrology social worker is a valuable resource for both HHD patients and care partners. This person has a unique role in providing support and assistance necessary to meet patients' logistical, monetary, emotional, and psychological needs. The social worker performs statutory duties and responsibilities per the CfC, including assessments for at-home risk, community care needs, and care partner needs. The social worker often coordinates home dialysis education and referral of interested in-center HD patients. Before initiating a patient on HHD, it may be wise to interview the patient and care partner separately to assess each individual's understanding and expectations of HHD. The technique failure rate for HHD in the initial 6 months (for nonmedical reasons) is quite high—managing patient expectations as well as identifying and addressing issues as early as possible may help to ensure success. Both patients and care partners should be encouraged to contact the social worker for support at any time. The responsibilities of the social worker also include assessing patients and care partners for burnout and need for respite. The social worker is also often involved in making arrangements for dialysis during planned travel.

Dietitian

The dietitian must be very knowledgeable about nutritional issues in HD, including the impact of HHD on nutrient management. HHD patients may require very different nutritional advice depending on their HHD prescription. For example, some patients on intensive HHD may require increased phosphorus and potassium intake. Ideally, the dietitian will interact with patients along with the multidisciplinary team during the monthly clinic visit, although in many instances the dietitian also covers large center-based HD programs and may not always be available at the home dialysis clinic.

Biomedical Technician

A biomedical dialysis technician may assist with installation and maintenance of HHD equipment and provide technical support. The quality of the dialysis delivered at home must meet the same specifications as center-based HD. Necessary skills include knowledge of equipment maintenance and water quality issues with HHD, participation in on-call service, and ability to perform home assessments and modifications to patient's dwellings to accommodate HHD. The ability to interact with patients and work with interdisciplinary staff can positively impact patients' experiences with HHD. Close collaboration and liaison with equipment vendors are necessary—many initial inquiries from a patient may be routed to the manufacturer's technical support department. Although many HHD centers have technicians on staff, some may contract with a dialysis machine vendor to provide technical support.

Administrative Support

One person is usually responsible for providing logistical support for the dialysis center (e.g., clinic scheduling, telephone triage, laboratory management, inventory, supply management, supply delivery, invoices, and billing support). Often he/she will act as the central coordinator of operations and, therefore, will need to communicate and maintain close links with staff, physicians, and patients. This person is frequently cross-trained as a dialysis technician, medical assistant, or phlebotomist to maximize efficiency. If these roles are left to the nursing staff, the efficiency of the clinic may lag.

Physician Education

The lack of vigorous nephrology home dialysis education and experience has been postulated to be one of the barriers to successful home dialysis. The American Society of Nephrology (ASN), in collaboration with George Washington University, publishes an annual survey on graduating trainees' assessment of their nephrology training. In a recent survey study, 41.4% and 61.7% of respondents indicated that they received little or no training on PD and HHD, respectively.[11] Only 55.6% of respondents ranked themselves as well trained and competent in the care of chronic PD patients; fewer perceived themselves as sufficiently trained for the care of self-care HD patients (33.8%) and HHD patients (15.8%). Most respondents believed these topics were relevant to their ultimate nephrology practice and desired more training during fellowship. Similar findings have been published elsewhere.[7] Given these perceived training deficits, the medical director of a home dialysis program will likely need to facilitate advanced HHD education of the nephrologists in the program (Table 15-2).

Table 15-2 PHYSICIAN EDUCATION RESOURCES

Meetings

Home Dialysis University
https://digital.lenos.com/northpointe/HDUFellows/
Hemodialysis University by ISHD and IU
http://www.ishd.org/meetings-hdu/
National Kidney Foundation
https://www.kidney.org/spring-clinical
Advance Renal Education Program
https://www.advancedrenaleducation.com/
Annual Dialysis Conference
https://annualdialysisconference.org/

Online resources

Renal Fellow Network
https://www.renalfellow.org/
ASN Online Curricula: Dialysis "Virtual Mentor"
https://www.asn-online.org/education/distancelearning/curricula/dialysis/
NephJC
http://www.nephjc.com/
UptoDate
https://www.uptodate.com/home
Home Dialysis Central
https://homedialysis.org/

TRAINING

HHD training is very time-consuming for both the patient and nurse, and represents a substantial economic investment for the dialysis provider. CMS recognizes this and provides additional training payments for 22 HHD sessions, Medicare eligibility on day 1 of HHD training, and a $500 training payment to the nephrologist. Typically, HHD training occurs 4 to 5 days per week for approximately 4 weeks with dialysis received during the training sessions. Often, even patients that will ultimately perform three times a week HHD will still train more frequently to improve knowledge retention and shorten overall training time. A regimented program is typically followed with tasks to be completed each week (Table 15-3).

It is essential to outline the schedule with expectations and responsibilities before initiating training. Adult learning principles should be

Table 15-3 TYPICAL HHD TRAINING PROGRAM	
Sample HHD Training Plan	
Week 1	• Infection control/Aseptic technique • HHD prescription • Cannulation • Machine setup
Week 2	• Managing medical complications • Troubleshooting alarms • Medication administration • Hazardous waste disposal
Week 3	• Obtaining lab specimens • Documenting treatments • Emergency/Disaster plans • Coping strategies for success at home
Week 4	• Patient and/or care partner independent practice • Supply management • Equipment maintenance

Source: Courtesy of Michelle Carver, RN.

followed as patients learn differently—use of auditory, tactile, kinesthetic, and visual techniques may be considered. The program should be tailored to support individual learning styles and speeds. Visual training aids that contain step-by-step photographs to demonstrate the dialysis procedure with a minimal amount of text may improve understanding. Feedback and repetition with testing following a training milestone should be considered to assess competence.

Educators often mistakenly perceive older patients as less willing to consider HHD. Motivation, comorbidities, physical and mental capacity, and the extra physical effort needed to conduct home dialysis may play varying roles in an older individual's decision and ability to undertake this modality.[12]

Various possibilities for training locations should be discussed to suit the learning demands of the individual. The training unit may be appropriate as it has the capability of running clinics, equipment demonstrations, and support for the trainer to educate multiple trainees at a time. However, there may be occasions when training in the home is more effective.

Even if the training is not done at home, home visits must be made prior and after completion of training to verify safety and suitability for HHD.

These visits ensure that setup and procedures used for training align with the particular physical arrangements at home. Most centers have the last training day in the patient's home.

[For more information, see Chapters 2, 13, and 14.]

■ CLINIC VISITS

CfC mandate monthly visits for home dialysis patients. In January 2019, visits for 2 of 3 consecutive months were permitted to be conducted by telehealth. The rapid implementation of telehealth for home dialysis in response to the COVID-19 coronavirus pandemic spurred the widespread use of telehealth, which could have a lasting impact on the management of HHD patients. Within weeks of social distancing guidelines being issued in 2020, a large percentage of HHD patients were utilizing telehealth visits rather than being seen in-person in the clinic.

An outline of typical tasks done at the monthly clinic visit are listed in Table 15-4; however, the visit should generally cover routine matters as critical issues regarding patient care should have been addressed already during the month.[1] Further, clinic staff should discuss any significant concerns with the physician before the visit to ensure visits are efficient. The critical portions of the monthly HHD visit are an examination of the vascular access, assessment of target weight, discussing patient-derived questions, and setting goals and targets for the upcoming month.

The patient experience is an essential aspect of dialysis treatment in the recent era of patient-oriented quality healthcare. Patient satisfaction with care correlates with perception of the quality of life and burden of illness, as well as improved intermediate outcomes in in-center HD patients.[13,14] Most patients spend 3 to 4 hours on HHD days setting up the machine and managing their dialysis, and go to the clinic for one to two clinic visits a month. Practices inattentive to wait times and other patient frustrations could potentially lose more than half of their patients each year and potential patients who hear of such inconveniences may be dissuaded from the clinic or the modality.[15]

The physical space guides the clinic flow. The multidisciplinary team may see the patient together in the room, or each team member may see the patient separately and communicate any issues after the visit. For detailed or sensitive conversations, a conference room may be suitable for maintaining the clinic flow and ensuring timely patient care. At the end of the visit, summarizing the discussions and setting goals improve patients' understanding. Contrary to perception, studies report that primary care providers (PCPs) remain involved in the care of the majority of

Table 15-4 KEY COMPONENTS OF MONTHLY CLINIC VISIT	
Treatment data	Pre and posttreatment vital signs Daily weights Access pressures Blood flow rate Ultrafiltration Adherence Machine alarms Prescription review
Supplies	Needles Dialysis medications Disposables Fluid bags Other medication refills
Access assessment	Physical exam Review of aseptic technique Review of cannulation method Needle site spacing Time to hemostasis Venous pressure review
Laboratory	Process samples (if brought from home) Draw needed samples (if not done) Review current labs Discuss previous labs (if needed)
On-site medicine administration	Intravenous iron Erythropoietin-stimulating agents Vaccines
Patient education	Access aseptic technique Machine setup Fluid removal Other topics (as needed)
Social situation assessment	Home environment Family support Vocational rehabilitation
Evaluation for care partner burnout	Need for respite care Discussion with social worker
Kidney transplantation	Referral Status Potential living donors

dialysis patients with an average of 4.5 primary care visits per patient-year at risk.[16] A collaborative care approach involving the PCPs may result in improved satisfaction.

[For more information, see Chapter 16.]

PATIENT AND CARE PARTNER BURNOUT

In the United States, discontinuation of HHD has been one of the significant contributors to the low prevalence of HHD for the past 50 years.[1] Technique failure, defined as discontinuation of HHD therapy, approaches 40% during the first 12 months of HHD in the United States.[17] Given the significant time commitment, infrastructure cost, and emotional investment associated with HHD training and initiation, technique failure has a detrimental impact on both facilities, staff, and patients. The chances of HHD technique failure increase with decreasing patient involvement in their care (e.g., setting up the machine, ordering supplies, arranging medications, cannulation, etc.). Race, ethnicity, and underlying cause of ESKD have not been associated with technique failure.[18] Interestingly, freedom from the dialysis center, uniformly seen in a positive manner by medical personnel, may provoke fear of isolation among families, spouses, and significant others, and could add to burnout and even depression. Offering respite care, a break from dialyzing at home with the direct supervision of staff, is a tool for addressing burnout.

[For more information, see Chapters 7 and 8.]

QUALITY ASSURANCE AND QUALITY IMPROVEMENT

Quality in healthcare has been an area of rising interest, with attempts to define quality and tie payment to the achievement of certain targets.[19] The Medicare Improvements for Patients and Providers Act (MIPPA) of 2008 created the End-Stage Renal Disease Prospective Payment System (PPS).[5] The PPS, which went into effect on January 1, 2011, includes a payment reduction if specific metrics are unmet. The program intends to promote high-quality care in outpatient dialysis facilities. Subsequently, dialysis facilities not meeting the standards in a calendar year (performance year) are subject to a global Medicare payment reduction of up to 2%.[20]

Dialysis Facility Compare (DFC) is a publicly accessible website that reports quality data on every Medicare-certified outpatient dialysis facility annually.[21] Some of the metrics intersect with PPS standards. DFC is a one to five "star" rating for each dialysis facility and must be displayed in the facility. Quality assurance (QA) is defined as monitoring of process and outcomes of care by review of medical records and predefined quality metrics as the End-Stage Renal Disease Quality Incentive Program (ESRD QIP) score and DFC star system. QAPI meetings and State surveys are tools for QA. State survey agencies perform QA to require facilities to meet minimum standards of operation to prevent. QAPI meetings should occur monthly and include representatives from all disciplines. Frequent review, with trending of outcomes and development of improvement plans when indicated, must be demonstrated. Table 15-5 shows a typical QAPI meeting agenda.[22]

Most nephrologists intend to provide high-quality care but may fall short due to limited training in QAPI processes during nephrology fellowship.[23] Root cause analysis is a basic component of QA. This type of analysis determines the most fundamental cause of an outcome and classifies it as infrastructure, process, or human.[24] The multidisciplinary team develops a plan for improvement while monitoring results. The Plan-Do-Study-Act cycle of quality improvement is then set into motion: set a realistic goal; layout a plan; execute it; reassess; and, depending on the outcome, modify or implement the process. This approach allows the facility to correct any identified problems that threaten the health and safety of patients, as mandated by the CfC. Maintenance and monitoring of quality of care is not only mandated but also crucial for patient-centric care.

[For more information, see Chapter 6.]

▌ECONOMICS OF HOME HEMODIALYSIS

Even the best HHD program cannot survive if it is not economically viable. The viability of any program depends on maximization of revenue and minimization of costs. The main difference between center-based HD and HHD are the higher labor and fixed capital costs of maintaining the HD center and the higher supply and training costs of HHD. However, there are several other considerations. Most HHD programs have fewer than 20 patients, and require at least one nurse. Thus, the labor costs for small HHD programs can be substantial. Home dialysis tends to attract roughly 2.5 times the number of patients with non-Medicare insurance, which currently pays substantially more for dialysis therapy than Medicare. Training HHD patients is associated with a high up-front cost. Most HHD programs will co-mingle resources and support with PD programs. Therefore, the most economically viable HHD programs are those that are larger, conducive to patients with commercial insurance, have low

Table 15-5   TYPICAL QAPI AGENDA FOR HHD PROGRAM
Monthly census and staffing ratios
Admissions, discharges, and training episodes
Hospitalization review • Reasons for admission
Bloodstream infections • Root cause analysis • Revolving episodes per 1000 treatment days rate
Review of urea kinetics
Anemia treatment outcomes
Bone and mineral disease treatment outcomes
Nutritional outcomes
Patient grievances and complaints
Transplantation review

"controllable" patient losses (<1% per month), and are associated with a vibrant PD program.

Analysis of the economics of the HHD program is done using a "cost per treatment" methodology. Involving all members of the HHD team in a review of such analysis may lead to the identification of opportunities to reduce costs (e.g., supply use). Figure 15-1 is an illustration of this methodology.

[For more information, see Chapter 14.]

▌ROLE OF TRANSITIONAL CARE UNITS

In most large practices, approximately half of dialysis initiation occurs in an unplanned, urgent, or emergent fashion, often in the inpatient setting. These new dialysis patients are at high risk for early morbidity and mortality as well as hospital readmission. Substantial education and discussion of dialysis options is often not provided and modality choice is limited. A transitional care unit (TCU) may make the transition to ESKD easier by providing more frequent dialysis sessions, focused and enhanced team interaction, patient-centered education, and adoption of a patient-preferred dialysis modality over an approximately 4-week period. By

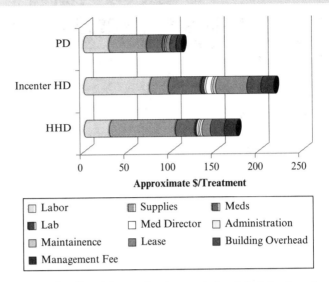

Figure 15-1 • Example of breakdown of various costs for dialysis treatments.

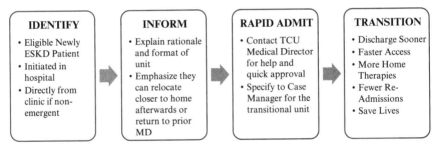

Figure 15-2 • Blueprint of transitional care unit workflow. *(Courtesy of Christopher Meshberger, MD.)*

providing additional focused outpatient care, it decreases dependency on the initial hospital setting as well as potentially improving patient outcomes during the incident ESKD period.[25]

TCUs can be located within the in-center HD unit, combined with a home dialysis facility, or exist as a separate stand-alone center. A separate physical area, dedicated and specifically trained staff, and allocation of additional resources—intensify the focus on the patient and provide optimal initiation of dialysis. A typical TCU workflow is outlined in Figure 15-2. The initial step is prescribing an individualized dialysis prescription, usually more frequent than thrice-weekly, to ensure clinical stability, resolution of uremic symptoms, prompt normalization of metabolic parameters, and control extracellular volume.

The duration of time in the TCU varies from person to person. After starting dialysis in a TCU, many patients will choose a home modality; thus, home dialysis education is a cornerstone of the TCU. The education that is provided encompasses psychological, lifestyle, nutritional, economic, vascular access, and dialysis modality topics.

▌ REFERENCES

1. Blagg CR, Hickman RO, Eschbach JW, Scribner BH. Home hemodialysis: six years' experience. *N Engl J Med.* 1970;283(21):1126-1131.
2. Blagg CR. The early history of dialysis for chronic renal failure in the United States: a view from Seattle. *Am J Kidney Dis.* 2007;49(3):482-496.
3. Berns JS. Training nephrology fellows in temporary hemodialysis catheter placement and kidney biopsies is needed and should be required. *Clin J Am Soc Nephrol.* 2018;13(7):1099-1101.
4. Rope RW, Pivert KA, Parker MG, Sozio SM, Merell SB. Education in nephrology fellowship: a survey-based needs assessment. *J Am Soc Nephrol.* 2017;28(7):1983-1990.
5. Department of Health and Human Services. Medicare and Medicaid programs: conditions for coverage of end-stage renal disease facilities. April 15, 2008. Available at https://www.cms.gov/Regulations-and-Guidance/Legislation/CFCsAndCoPs/downloads/ESRDfinalrule0415.pdf. Accessed September 20, 2019.
6. ESRD QIP summary: payment years 2016-2020. Available at https://www.cms.gov/Medicare/Quality-Initiatives-Patient-Assessment-Instruments/ESRDQIP/Downloads/ESRD-QIP-Summary-Payment-Years-2016---2020.pdf. Accessed September 20, 2019.
7. O'Hare AM, Johansen KL, Rodriguez RA. Dialysis and kidney transplantation among patients living in rural areas of the United States. *Kidney Int.* 2006;69(2):343-349.
8. Prakash S, Coffin R, Schold J, et al. Travel distance and home dialysis rates in the United States. *Perit Dial Int.* 2014;34(1):24-32.
9. Wallace EL GR, Koenig KL, Crain LA Regional impact of geography on home dialysis utilization. *J Nephrol Ther.* 2014;4(176). doi:10.4172/2161-0959.1000176.
10. Rastogi A, Chertow GM. Mandating staffing ratios in hemodialysis facilities: California SB 349 and unintended consequences. *Clin J Am Soc Nephrol.* 2018;13(7):1110-1112.
11. Parker MG, Ibrahim T, Shaffer R, Rosner MH, Molitoris BA. The future nephrology workforce: will there be one? *Clin J Am Soc Nephrol.* 2011;6(6):1501-1506.
12. Pipkin M, Eggers PW, Larive B, et al. Recruitment and training for home hemodialysis: experience and lessons from the Nocturnal Dialysis Trial. *Clin J Am Soc Nephrol.* 2010;5(9):1614-1620.

13. Kimmel PL. Psychosocial factors in adult end-stage renal disease patients treated with hemodialysis: correlates and outcomes. *Am J Kidney Dis.* 2000;35(4 suppl 1):S132-S140.

14. Kimmel PL, Peterson RA, Weihs KL, et al. Multiple measurements of depression predict mortality in a longitudinal study of chronic hemodialysis outpatients. *Kidney Int.* 2000;57(5):2093-2098.

15. Practices must reduce patient wait times—here's how. Available at https://www.softwareadvice.com/resources/reducing-patient-wait-times/. Accessed October 4, 2019.

16. Thorsteinsdottir B, Ramar P, Hickson LJ, et al. Care of the dialysis patient: primary provider involvement and resource utilization patterns—a cohort study. *BMC Nephrol.* 2017;18(1):322.

17. Weinhandl ED, Nieman KM, Gilbertson DT, Collins AJ. Hospitalization in daily home hemodialysis and matched thrice-weekly in-center hemodialysis patients. *Am J Kidney Dis.* 2015;65(1):98-108.

18. Pauly RP, Rosychuk RJ, Usman I, et al. Technique failure in a multicenter Canadian home hemodialysis cohort. *Am J Kidney Dis.* 2019;73(2):230-239.

19. Donabedian A. Evaluating the quality of medical care. 1966. *Milbank Q.* 2005;83(4):691-729. doi:10.1111/j.1468-0009.2005.00397.x.

20. Gupta N, Wish JB. Do current quality measures truly reflect the quality of dialysis? *Semin Dial.* 2018;31(4):406-414.

21. Fishbane S, Hazzan A. Meeting the 2012 QIP (Quality Incentive Program) clinical measures: strategies for dialysis centers. *Am J Kidney Dis.* 2012;60(5 suppl 1): S5-S13; quiz S14-S17.

22. Conditions for Coverage (CfCs) & Conditions of Participations (CoPs) condition for coverage. Available at https://www.cms.gov/Regulations-and-Guidance/Legislation/CFCsAndCoPs/index.html. Accessed July 9, 2019.

23. Prince LK, Little DJ, Schexneider KI, Yuan CM. Integrating quality improvement education into the nephrology curricular milestones framework and the clinical learning environment review. *Clin J Am Soc Nephrol.* 2017;12(2):349-356.

24. Charles R, Hood B, Derosier JM, et al. How to perform a root cause analysis for workup and future prevention of medical errors: a review. *Patient Saf Surg.* 2016;10:20.

25. Bowman B, Zheng S, Yang A, et al. Improving incident ESRD care via a transitional care unit. *Am J Kidney Dis.* 2018;72(2):278-283.

REMOTE MONITORING AND HOME HEMODIALYSIS

16

Danielle Wentworth and Emaad M. Abdel-Rahman

Patients with end-stage kidney disease (ESKD) undergoing home hemodialysis (HHD) make up only a small fraction of all patients receiving renal replacement therapy (RRT) in the United States. According to the United States Renal Data System (USRDS), there were 106,915 incident in-center hemodialysis (HD) patients (88.5% of all incident dialysis patients) compared to only 488 HHD patients (0.4%) in 2017.[1] Among prevalent patients at the end of 2017, there were 458,125 in-center HD patients (87.5%) and only 9460 HHD patients (1.8%), with the remainder of ESKD patients utilizing peritoneal dialysis (PD) or undergoing renal transplant.[1] Given the low utilization of HHD, there has been significant interest in identifying the barriers that preclude greater use of this treatment modality. Some of the most prominent factors include patient and/or care partner misconceptions about level of difficulty, lack of confidence in performing HHD, concerns about troubleshooting issues that arise during home therapy, and feelings of isolation from medical providers.[2] However, the overall risks to patients undergoing HHD are very low, with one study citing a procedure-related adverse event rate of 0.06 per 1000 HHD treatments, and overall death rate of 0.0085 per 1000 treatments.[3]

In August 2017, the NxStage System One dialysis device was approved by the United States Food and Drug Administration (FDA) for solo HHD during a patient's waking hours.[4] This expanded access to HHD to patients who wish to dialyze without a care partner. Currently, there is no published data on the safety and efficacy of solo HHD. In an analysis of 117,000 HHD treatments, Wong and colleagues examined seven reported adverse events. They noted that five of the seven reported adverse events were related to human error and poor protocol adherence, and two of those seven patients had been dialyzing alone at the time of the incident. For patients undergoing HHD, whether with a care partner or solo, having remote access to a healthcare provider may help alleviate concerns about having to manage problems that arise on their own.[3] Telemedicine offers services specifically designed to assist patients, care partners, and their medical dialysis team to address these concerns.

The American Telemedicine Association defines telemedicine as "the use of medical information exchanged from one site to another via electronic communication to improve patients' health status."[5] Telehealth refers to a broader range of health-related services such as education, remote monitoring, and provider-to-provider consultation, in addition to patient care. Telehealth can occur via several modalities, which include real-time telemedicine, store-and-forward telemedicine, remote patient monitoring (RPM), and the use of mobile health services supported by mobile communication devices, such as wireless patient monitoring devices, smartphones, personal digital assistants, and tablet computers. For real-time telemedicine, the patient and/or surrogate interacts with the healthcare provider through audiovisual technology. Store-and-forward telemedicine involves the electronic transmission of recorded medical information through secure portals. Finally, RPM collects a patient's medical data then transmits it to a healthcare provider at a remote location. For this chapter, we will focus on direct patient care through telemedicine.

In order to understand how telemedicine can specifically benefit patients undergoing HHD, it is first important to understand how these technologies have evolved for this particular ESKD modality.

BRIEF HISTORY OF TELEMEDICINE AND HOME HEMODIALYSIS

Utilizing telemedicine for patients undergoing HHD is not a novel idea. As early as the 1970s, RPM systems were developed to record patient information during HHD treatments as well as monitor machines and alarms, with transmittal of data to a centralized, yet remote location.[6] Before the Internet, the data was transmitted via direct telephone lines. Unfortunately, RPM at the time was limited by the cost of using long-distance telephone lines, and the individual observing the incoming data was not able to immediately act upon any alarms received during the patient's treatment.[6]

With these limitations in mind, subsequent HHD programs determined that monitoring of intradialytic events in real-time was necessary. This was particularly true for nocturnal HHD programs, since their patients were often asleep and alone during treatment, and there was concern that a catastrophe could occur if monitoring was not available.[7] The first formal nocturnal HHD program was established in Toronto, Canada in 1994 by Uldall and colleagues, and they implemented their own RPM program to track patients.[6] For their initial RPM program, a modified Fresenius 2008H dialysis machine was monitored remotely via a modem connection. Software was installed on a patient's home computer so that it could transmit data from the HHD machine to a remote observer, who had to manually pull data, one home computer at a time, every few minutes during these overnight treatments.[8]

Shortly thereafter, Cybernius Medical Ltd. developed the DAX dialysis software, an RPM that was marketed for commercial availability. At the time, this software was unique, in that it was able to provide an observer data in real time from patients' HHD treatments and data was rapidly transmitted through a modem without the need to install additional software on a patient's home computer.[6,8] This feature allowed for an observer to receive live alarms from a patient's home machine; if the patient did not correct the alarm after a few minutes, the observer would call the patient through a secondary telephone line. Since these observers were not medical professionals, if they were unable to address the problem, they could then contact the patient's healthcare team member on-call.[8]

During the same time period, as part of the European Union Commission-funded HOME Rehabilitation Treatment-Dialysis Project, Skiadas and colleagues also investigated whether RPM could be used to help support HHD patients.[9] HD machines were installed in four hospital renal units. These dialysis machines were then modified so information could be transmitted via a network card and router over a bidirectional communication network line. During treatments, data such as blood pressure, pulse oximetry, heart rate, and electrocardiograms were transmitted to a central control station staffed with a nurse or physician. When a dialysis machine alarmed, this data was sent to the central control station to be acted upon by the staff member monitoring the treatment. Overall, they evaluated 305 HD sessions for 29 patients, and the RPM system worked as expected, delivering appropriate information to satellite observers who could then take action if necessary and communicate with the patient.

Despite these advances, early RPM systems were imperfect. For example, when an alarm went off during an HHD treatment and was transmitted to a remote observer, it was not always clear to that observer which patient's machine was the source of the alarm. Furthermore, the severity of alarms was not always distinguishable, so that an alarm notifying the remote observer about a blood leak or air detection in the blood would appear the same as an alarm notifying them about a breach in treatment parameters (such as blood pressure). Another concern was that the alarm and intervention information both had to be documented manually in flowsheets. In the early 2000s, Fresenius employed an RPM system to monitor up to 48 nocturnal HHD patients, staffed by two certified technicians. During just 1 month of monitoring with the DAX software, 571 HHD treatments were complicated by 76 patient alarms, ranging from blood pressure alarms (48 total) to one air detection.[6]

To address these original limitations, in the early 2000s, Fresenius developed the iCare Monitoring System for their 2008 series HHD machine, an RPM system that was able to prioritize the severity of alarms to centralized remote observers.[6,10] Furthermore, the system was able to automatically document alarms and their interventions, making it a much better tool for smaller HHD programs that could not previously afford RPM. The biggest downside to the iCare system was that it could be only used with Fresenius HD machines.

Today, despite a long history of RPM, real-time monitoring of patients undergoing HHD has fallen out of favor due to concerns over safety and cost-effectiveness, given the overall safety of HHD. Marshall and colleagues described that among 17 surveyed Canadian HHD programs, none were using real-time RPM at the time of the survey, and 82% of those programs had never utilized it at all.[7] While RPM did help patients new to HHD adjusting to their treatments in the first few months, its overall life-saving capabilities were limited: over 20 years of monitoring, one program only had two life-threatening episodes identified because of real-time monitoring.[7] Another center in Canada reported that their rate of life-threatening adverse events was only 9 per 1000 patient-years, which is comparable to outcomes for patients undergoing in-center HD.[7] Paying observers to monitor patients undergoing a treatment considered to be safe was not thought to be the best use of center funds, and dialysis programs decided to spend that money elsewhere.[7]

THE FUTURE FOR REMOTE PATIENT MONITORING AND TELEMEDICINE IN HOME HEMODIALYSIS

Although real-time RPM has fallen out of favor in the HHD community, there are recent technological advances that still help HHD patients connect to their providers remotely. Currently, NxStage Medical has its own proprietary telemedicine platform called the Nx2me Connected Health application (app) for use with the NxStage System One. With this platform, the company aims to decrease HHD technique failure and patient attrition.[11] Nx2me collects patient treatment data and can transmit that information to the patient's nephrology team to review after each treatment. However, unlike other forms of RPM, Nx2me transmits data after the patient's HHD treatment, and does not send alarms to a remote location. This telemedicine platform works by capturing information from the NxStage machine, sending that information to the Nx2me app, and then that data is sent through a secure server to the clinician portal. The app can collect information about a patient's weight, blood pressure, ultrafiltration rate and amount, medications taken during an HHD treatment, and the amount of dialysate delivered, and patients can also add comments about their treatments. Information can be transmitted either through a secure Wi-Fi network, or through a cellular network if Wi-Fi is unavailable. With their retrospective study about the Nx2me app, Weinhandl and Collins demonstrated that the program did help reduce attrition rates and technique failure, and that patients using the technology were more likely to complete their HHD training.[11]

In July of 2019, Fresenius Medical Care North America announced that they are working on a real-time, continuous RPM platform and had invested in a Denver-based company called BioIntelliSense, Inc.[12] Further details are currently unavailable, and the target population for the RPM platform is not clear at this time.

While the future for real-time RPM in HHD is unclear, there have been recent legislative changes in the United States that have brought telemedicine back into the spotlight for patients undergoing HHD.

❚ LEGISLATION AND POLICIES IN THE UNITED STATES

In February 2018, the 2018 Bipartisan Budget Act was passed, extending telemedicine benefits to Medicare beneficiaries undergoing home dialysis, including PD and HHD.[13] Starting January 1, 2019, patients undergoing HHD were granted the option to receive monthly care via telemedicine. Under current guidelines, patients may have two of three monthly visits every quarter conducted remotely. The exception to this is new patients, whose first three monthly visits after initiating HHD must be done face-to-face.[14] Before this Act was signed, telemedicine encounters were limited by restrictions concerning originating sites, distant site practitioners, and specific telemedicine and telehealth services.[13]

Originating Sites

To conduct a telemedicine visit, the patient must be at an originating site. Medicare defines an originating site as a specific location where a Medicare beneficiary receives telehealth services. Examples of originating sites include a provider's clinic, hospitals, federally qualified health centers, skilled nursing facilities, dialysis facilities, and most important for HHD patients, the homes of patients with ESKD undergoing home dialysis.[15] Prior to 2019, originating sites could not include a home dialysis patient's home or a nonhospital-based dialysis facility.

Distant Site Practitioners

A distant site practitioner is a provider that is able to furnish telemedicine services. State law specifies which providers are covered for telemedicine encounters, but the category includes physicians, physician assistants, advanced-practice nurses, clinical psychologists, social workers, and registered dietitians.[15] Additionally, the practitioner must be licensed in the state of the patient's originating site. For example, if a physician licensed in Virginia is providing telemedicine services to a patient living in Tennessee, that patient would need to conduct their visit from a Virginia originating site. Furthermore, it is important for the practitioner to ensure that they are properly credentialed at the patient's originating site, unless the site is the patient's home if they are undergoing a home dialysis modality. Practitioners should also ensure that their malpractice insurance covers telemedicine encounters and services. Finally, for practitioners documenting a telemedicine encounter, it is important to include a "Telemedicine Disclaimer" in the patient's progress notes.[13]

Telemedicine Services

In order to conduct a telemedicine visit, the distant site practitioner and patient (at the originating site) must utilize real-time interactive audio and visual telecommunication.[15] For HHD patients, equipment for telemedicine visits from their home should include access to broadband Internet with a connection that is fast enough to enable transfer of audio and visual data, a Health Insurance Portability and Accountability Act (HIPAA)-compliant webcam or mobile device camera for video conferencing, and a digital stethoscope for physical examination. During the telemedicine visit, a nonmedically trained care partner can facilitate the visit as a clinical presenter, placing the digital stethoscope in the correct locations as directed by the distant site practitioner. Alternatively, clinical presenters can, with 2 to 3 hours of training, act as the patient's telemedicine visit facilitator.[13]

❚ BENEFITS OF TELEMEDICINE

With changing technology and legislative policies, telemedicine will undoubtedly play a larger role in the management of HHD patients going forward. Keeping this in mind, it is important to realize that while telemedicine has multiple benefits for patients, care partners, and healthcare providers, there can also be challenges with its implementation (Table 16-1).

Travel and Time

With the recent guidelines allowing remote visits in place of a face-to-face visits 2 out of every 3 months, travel time for patients should decrease.[16] This decrease in travel time is not only helpful for patients who live in rural areas, but also for those traveling from suburban and urban areas, who may feel burdened dealing with traffic, parking, and public transportation.[14] For providers, providing two monthly visits every quarter via telemedicine helps minimize the amount of traveling required between units, especially for providers working in less densely populated areas.

Decreasing travel time to and from a dialysis unit will help save patients and care partners' time and money.

Patient Access

With the development of newer technologies, a full clinical examination can be performed on HHD patients remotely. A full remote visit still allows the healthcare provider and multidisciplinary dialysis team to interact with patients via a two-way audiovisual system, and also allows for patients to have easier access to their providers. This has the potential to enable the team to provide better medical and psychological support to their patients. Furthermore, this increased access to providers may help identify any developing problems sooner, thus allowing earlier intervention and problem solving.[13]

Cost Savings

Compared to face-to-face visits, Ehrlich and colleagues showed an annual cost savings of approximately $5000/year when patient visits were conducted remotely by telemedicine, without any change in outcomes.[17]

Patient Satisfaction

Several small studies have shown that HHD patient satisfaction has improved with the use of telemedicine.[18–20] For instance, telemedicine can provide a greater sense of security for patients.[20] This increased patient satisfaction with HHD, as well as the extended healthcare services to rural and isolated communities that can be offered by telemedicine, has the potential to increase the number of patients choosing this modality.

▌CHALLENGES WITH THE USE OF TELEMEDICINE

Despite all of the benefits, use of telemedicine in the care of HHD patients also has its challenges (Table 16-1). Challenges to the use of telemedicine can be divided into the following.

Patient Issues

While HHD patients have easier access to providers with telemedicine, some patients may feel more isolated and anxious about being at home without regular in-person visits. Some may have a sense of being abandoned. Additionally, patients may still need to travel to their dialysis units to have monthly bloodwork drawn and to obtain their dialysis-related medications and supplies, leaving them with a travel burden nonetheless.[14]

Provider Issues

Despite advanced technology offering varying methods to perform physical examination remotely, the healthcare provider may face challenges assessing volume status and the dialysis access. Furthermore, some providers may miss having in-person patient interactions. Fewer face-to-face patient-provider interactions could further contribute to provider burnout and dissatisfaction.[14]

Table 16-1 BENEFITS AND CHALLENGES OF TELEMEDICINE	
Benefits	**Challenges**
Patient convenience	*Patient issues*
• Reduces/Eliminates travel and saves time	• Patients may feel isolated, abandoned, or anxious about being at home without regular in-person visits
Patient access	*Provider issues*
• Increased access to healthcare services: extend nephrology consultation to rural and isolated communities	• Many providers prefer in-person patient interactions and fewer face-to-face patient-provider interactions could further provider burnout and dissatisfaction
• Enhanced access to specialists: Nephrologist coordination and education to PCP/patients	
• Reduced hospitalizations/ER visits	• Inability to fully examine patients, including physical evaluation of volume status and the dialysis access
• Increase home dialysis volume→ more market share	*Ethical issues*
• Providers may gain valuable insight into the home environment of home dialysis patients without home-visit	• Equity, privacy, confidentiality, and informed consent
Cost savings	*Financial issues*
• Cost-effective method of service delivery, no facility fees charged	• Half of US smartphone users with no other access to the Internet had to cancel/shut off their cell phone service due to financial concerns
Patient satisfaction	*Technical difficulties*
• Improved quality of care	• Limited access to equipment, loss of signals
• Allow providers to spend more time with the patient during telehealth encounters→ patient and provider satisfaction	*Administrative issues*
	• Need for credentialing, licensure, and front-end investments

Ethical Issues

Telemedicine may be associated with considerable concern pertaining to patients' confidentiality and privacy. Additionally, some patients may lack the infrastructure supporting telemedicine, thus contributing to biased and unequal opportunity offered to patients.[13,14]

Financial Issues

While telemedicine may be cost-saving due to reduced travel to dialysis centers, some patients' ability to utilize telemedicine may be limited by other financial concerns. Some patients may not have access to the Internet beyond a smartphone, and patients may need to cancel/shut off their cell phone service for a period of time due to financial instability.[21]

From a program standpoint, there is also a need for front-end investment to have the necessary infrastructure in place.[14] In addition, implementation of different telehealth technologies will require training of providers and patients at an added expense.[13]

Technical Difficulties

Some patients may have limited access to the needed equipment or limited remote connectivity, complicating telehealth visits.[14,19] For example, Minatodani and colleagues reported that 27.3% of patients in their nurse-driven telehealth monitoring study experienced technical difficulties.[19] Additionally, poorly designed telehealth platforms can lead to frustration for both patients and providers and also result in poor quality visits.[14]

Administrative Issues

There are multiple regulatory issues that must be addressed, such as credentialing, licensure, malpractice insurance coverage, and reimbursement for services for non-Medicare beneficiaries.[13]

Sustainability

Once a telemedicine program is established, measures must be taken to ensure its sustainability. In the iNephro study, the investigators distributed a free smartphone application to German-speaking chronic kidney disease patients to assist them in medication adherence and documentation of blood pressure. After 11,688 smartphone users downloaded the application and demonstrated initial engagement, a significant drop-off in the use of the application was reported at 2 months with less than 1% using the application at least weekly 1 year after download.[22]

Telemedicine has developed and advanced in recent years. The new guidelines extending telemedicine benefits to patients on home dialysis have opened the door for further use of this technology to better care of these patients. Data on outcomes associated with the use of telemedicine in patients with kidney disease on HHD is lacking and large randomized trials are needed to further our knowledge base.

▌REFERENCES

1. United States Renal Data System. 2018 ADR reference tables: treatment modalities. United States Renal Data System. Available at https://www.usrds.org/reference.aspx. Accessed March 25, 2020.

2. Walker RC, Howard K, Morton RL. Home hemodialysis: a comprehensive review of patient-centered and economic considerations. *Clinicoecon Outcomes Res.* 2017;9:149-161.

3. Wong B, Zimmerman D, Reintjes F, et al. Procedure-related serious adverse events among home hemodialysis patients: a quality assurance perspective. *Am J Kidney Dis.* 2014;63(2):251-258.

4. U.S. Food and Drug Administration. Traditional 510(k) premarket notification. Available at https://www.accessdata.fda.gov/cdrh_docs/pdf17/K171331.pdf. Published August 24, 2017. Accessed October 1, 2019.

5. American Telemedicine Association. Telemedicine glossary. Available at https://thesource.americantelemed.org/resources/telemedicine-glossary. Accessed October 1, 2019.

6. Diaz-Buxo JA, Schlaeper C, Van Valkenburgh D. Evolution of home hemodialysis monitoring systems. *Hemodial Int.* 2003;7(4):35.

7. Marshall MR, Pierratos A, Pauly RP. Delivering home hemodialysis: is there still a role for real-time treatment monitoring? *Semin Dial.* 2015;28(2):176-179.

8. Pierratos A, Ouwendyk M, Francoeur R, et al. Nocturnal hemodialysis: three-year experience. *J Am Soc Nephrol.* 1998;9(5):859-868.

9. Skiadas M, Agroyiannis B, Carson E, et al. Design, implementation and preliminary evaluation of a telemedicine system for home haemodialysis. *J Telemed Telecare.* 2002;8(3):157-164.

10. Schlaeper C, Diaz-Buxo JA. The Fresenius Medical Care home hemodialysis system. *Semin Dial.* 2004;17(2):159-161.

11. Weinhandl ED, Collins AJ. Relative risk of home hemodialysis attrition in patients using a telehealth platform. *Hemodial Int.* 2018;22(3):318-327.

12. Fresenius Medical Care. Fresenius Medical Care North America invests in remote patient monitoring. Available at https://fmcna.com/news/news-releases/fresenius-medical-care-north-america-invests-in-biointellisense-/. Published July 9, 2019. Accessed October 1, 2019.

13. Lew SQ, Sikka N. Operationalizing telehealth for home dialysis patients in the United States. *Am J Kidney Dis.* 2019;74(1):95-100.
14. Bieber SD, Weiner DE. Telehealth and home dialysis: a new option for patients in the United States. *Clin J Am Soc Nephrol.* 2018;13(8):1288-1290.
15. Centers for Medicare & Medicaid Services: telehealth services. Available at https://www.cms.gov/Outreach-and-Education/Medicare-Learning-Network-MLN/MLNProducts/downloads/TelehealthSrvcsfctsht.pdf. Published January 2019. Accessed October 1, 2019.
16. H.R. 1892—Bipartisan Budget Act of 2018 Section 50302—Expanding access to home dialysis therapy. Available at https://www.congress.gov/115/bills/hr1892/BILLS-115hr1892enr.pdf. Accessed March 29, 2020.
17. Ehrlich J, Neuberger ML, Hofmann M, Brophy P, Nester CM. Remote access using Skype. Annual Dialysis Conference Abstract, Georgia World Congress Center, Atlanta, GA, 2014.
18. Whitten P, Buis L. Use of telemedicine for haemodialysis: perceptions of patients and health-care providers, and clinical effects. *J Telemed Telecare.* 2008;14(2):75-78.
19. Minatodani DE, Chao PJ, Berman SJ. Home telehealth: facilitators, barriers, and impact of nurse support among high-risk dialysis patients. *Telemed J E Health.* 2013;19(8):573-578.
20. Rygh E, Arlid E, Johnsen E, Rumpsfeld M. Choosing to live with home dialysis—patient's experiences and potential for telemedicine support: a qualitative study. *BMC Nephrol.* 2012;13:13.
21. Smith A. U.S. smartphone use in 2015. Pew Research Center. Published April 1, 2015. Available at https://www.pewresearch.org/internet/2015/04/01/us-smartphone-use-in-2015/. Accessed October 12, 2019.
22. Becker S, Kribben A, Meister S, Diamantidis CJ, Unger N, Mitchell A. User profiles of a smartphone application to support drug adherence—experiences from the iNephro project. *PLoS One.* 2013;8(10):e78547.

Index

Page numbers followed by f or t indicate figures or tables, respectively.